THE
SPATIAL CHILD

THE
SPATIAL CHILD

By

JOHN PHILO DIXON, Ph.D.

Research Director
Center for Theater Techniques
in Education
American Shakespeare Theater
Stratford, Connecticut

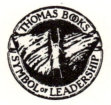

CHARLES C THOMAS • PUBLISHER
Springfield • Illinois • U.S.A.

Published and Distributed Throughout the World by

CHARLES C THOMAS • PUBLISHER

2600 South First Street

Springfield, Illinois 62717, U.S.A.

© *1983 by* CHARLES C THOMAS • PUBLISHER

ISBN 0-398-04821-5

Library of Congress Catalog Card Number: 83-386

With THOMAS BOOKS *careful attention is given to all details of manufacturing and
design. It is the Publisher's desire to present books that are satisfactory as to their physical
qualities and artistic possibilities and appropriate for their particular use.* THOMAS
BOOKS *will be true to those laws of quality that assure a good name and good will.*

Printed in the United States of America
CU-R-1

Library of Congress Cataloging in Publication Data

Dixon, John Philo.
  The spatial child.

  Bibliography: p.
  Includes index.
    1. Gifted children--Education.   2. Space perception.
I. Title.
LC3993.2.D48 1983   371.95′2   83-386
ISBN 0-398-04821-5

To Jane
  For all the encouragement

To Steven and Bonnie
  For being so special

He was last in the lowermost class but one. . . . Dull boys were now and then put over him in form.

From

> *Isaac Newton: A Biography*
> by Louis Trenchard More

There was no possibility of his passing an examination in any subject but drawing, no possibility at all.

From

> *Picasso: A Biography*
> by Patrick O'Brian

He seemed to be genuinely retarded. His dictation was riddled with crass spelling-mistakes. He never succeeded in learning Latin like the others, and his mathematics were non-existent.

From

> *Rodin*
> by Bernard Champigneulle

When Hermann Einstein asked his son's headmaster what profession his son should adopt, the answer was simply: "It doesn't matter; he'll never make a success of anything."

From

> *Einstein: The Life And Times*
> by Ronald W. Clark

PREFACE

RESEARCH on the nature of spatial ability has come such a long way in the last century that one would expect it to have considerable impact on the way educators understand giftedness in children. Yet, with few exceptions, when one looks at the spectrum of programs for gifted children, one senses that the accumulated knowledge on spatial ability has been given little if any consideration and has no impact on the planning of these programs. This book has been written for the purpose of addressing this shortcoming. Spatial ability is one of the primary ways in which giftedness is manifested in many children. We can hardly move forward in our understanding of giftedness until we have focused on the implications of this.

It is also my purpose to take up one particularly sticky issue with regard to spatial ability. Outstanding spatial ability often manifests itself in children who are mediocre, sometimes debilitated, in other important academic skills — most often in language skills. The cases of persons of historical genius who had a natural inclination toward spatial ability, but a deficiency in other academic skills, are so striking that they suggest we should more often than not look for spatial genius to be unrelated to more conspicuous academic skills. It should be considered an embarrassment to the weak conceptions of giftedness that prevail among educators that persons like Albert Einstein, Pablo Picasso, Auguste Rodin, Isaac Newton, and Niels Bohr would not fit with them.

This is a difficult issue indeed. It implies a direction completely contrary to the traditions from which the field of gifted education has emerged. Most children are labeled gifted either because they have distinguished themselves in standard school performance or because they have received a high score on a test of general intelligence or general creativity. The problem is that many children who possess great potential will not manifest their abilities in a standard academic way or on a test of general abilities. Their abilities are specialized in ways not amenable to recognition in the usual school setting. These children are rarely included in programs for the gifted or properly served when included. This is perhaps more the case with spatial ability than with any other area. Hopefully, a reading of this book will be convincing on this point.

In the attempt to make this case, I have had to roam a broad and varied territory; biographies, educational psychology, cognitive psychology, testing theories, the mathematics of factor analysis, neurology and neuropsychology, developmental psychology, learning theories, personality theories and research, education for the gifted, creativity research, and gestalt psychology. Few people achieve expertise in more than one of these fields. One roams the broad territory with considerable trepidation. It would have been more secure to work with a more circumscribed topic, or, to put it in Einstein's beautiful words of metaphoric derision, it might have been safer to "take a board of wood, look for its thinnest part, and drill a great number of holes where drilling is easy." However, gaining wisdom concerning a problem often requires approaching the problem from a variety of perspectives. One hopes the wisdom gained outweighs any deficiencies in dealing with the expanse of knowledge.

JPD

ACKNOWLEDGMENTS

FORTUNATELY I have been helped by others who have come this way before me, most notably British psychologist I. Mac-Farlane Smith and also American learning disabilities specialist Alexander Bannatyne. Those who have provided and shared information valuable to this book are Sunny Chang, E. Paul Torrance, Richard Sullivan, Abraham Tannenbaum, Linda Dubin, Lucile Beckman, Gene Glass, Sue Baum, Frances Karnes, Joan Hickey, Lee Walker, Sandra Black, Barbara Ryan, Jane Weber, Betty Peterson, Mary Fussell, Frances Bennett, Jean Blanning, Mogens Jensen, Walter Jones, Rosa Quezada, and Jack Gillette. Those who have given generously of their time in making this book possible are Mary Laycock, Peter and Catherine Jackson, and Patricia Moore. To Joe Renzulli must go both the blame and the thanks for getting me involved in such a fascinating field of study. Thanks also go to my colleagues at the Center For Theatre Techniques, Mary Hunter Wolf, Sharyn Esdaile, Sue Hill, Lynn Niro, and Keith Cunningham, for their patience while I was preoccupied with this task. While completing the manuscript, I have appreciated the interest and encouragement of Payne Thomas of Charles C Thomas, Publisher.

A special thanks to my mother for forbearance in helping me learn to read — without which writing would have been impossible. Finally, it is most important to say that my wife Jane was a partner in this effort from the inception of the book. Her encouragement and editorial assistance at every stage of the writing kept the book on track. If the book is readable, it is due to her efforts and willingness to take valuable time from her work at Yale University.

CONTENTS

THE
SPATIAL CHILD

SECTION I
UNDERSTANDING THE
SPATIAL CHILD

Chapter 1

THE SPATIAL CHILD

THE PROBLEM AS EXPERIENCED

IT was a combination of mystification and depression that set in when Mrs. Wilson struggled at introducing me to reading in the first grade. As I looked around at my classmates, their ease at turning written words into the correct spoken words seemed to make them coconspirators. They possessed a secret wisdom to which I was not privy. Mrs. Wilson looked upon them with eyes of pleasure. They were her teacher's delight, her measure of success. She looked upon me with eyes of forlorn patience. I was the stumbling block in her attempt to deliver a class full of readers to the second grade teachers. I remember sitting bent low at my school desk, eyes downward, hoping not to be noticed as I bumbled over *Dick and Jane*.

Panic struck me when my mother had to visit school to talk about my difficulties. My mother had never had doubts about me. I could run, I could talk, I could play games, I could build things, I could sing — all those things that mark normalcy to a hopeful mother. Mrs. Wilson had found me defective, and I had become a problem child, even to those who were most dear to me. My mother's visit to Mrs. Wilson also caused terror in the confusion of my child's mind. I feared that my unused schemes to cheat on spelling tests — a strategic planning undertaken in the desire to avoid being lowest in the class — might have been found out. Perhaps Mrs. Wilson in her infinite wisdom could even read into the hearts of little boys. However, the conference had only to do with my incompetence. My mother sat beside Mrs. Wilson, and I sat at my desk across the otherwise empty room. My ears strained to hear bits and pieces of the litany of my problems. Mrs. Wilson concluded that I wasn't prepared to go on to second grade. Flunking was the ultimate stigma for a school child in rural Nebraska. It would have put my self-regard at the lowest of levels. To my everlasting gratitude, things weren't left at that. A deal was struck between Mrs. Wilson and my mother. I would only be allowed to enter second grade in the fall if my mother gave me special instruction in reading for the whole summer vacation. My mother's reading lessons had little more effect than those of Mrs. Wilson. I tried, but reading wasn't yet in me.

I entered second grade as much a nonreader as before, but thanked my lucky stars that I had made it, and braced for another year of being the uninformed outsider in a society of secret code decipherers. Sometime during the second grade I began to catch on to reading, and I don't remember being in serious threat of flunking after that. My school performance settled into the slow-poke category for most of elementary school. There were a few breaks in this eight-year stint of questionable reputation. There was the day the second grade teacher asked several students to make a line a yard long on the chalkboard without looking at the yard stick. Mine came closest to being the right length. The teacher hardly noticed this insignificant victory of one of her more unpromising students, but for me it was one of those rare triumphs that stands etched in my mind.

My third grade teacher told my mother there was a lot going on in my mind. How did she guess? In the small town in which I grew up, the "farmerish" wisdom of silence would occasionally be applied to me; more than a few times people would take note of my basically unspoken character and say, "Still water runs deep." I never did know how to take that. Was deep good or bad?

There was the week in Miss Reine's fourth grade class. I was allowed to help construct a model colonial village. I made houses, a stockade, and an intricate little spinning wheel. It was the most glorious week in elementary school. As far as I was concerned, it could have gone on forever. However, then it was necessary to move on to the "real" work of school. Miss Reine told me that I couldn't work on the model any more because I had spent too much time and gotten behind in my school work.

Throughout these eight years there was an interesting discrepancy. Although my reading never changed from a slow to halting pace, I nevertheless loved reading. Sometimes I would spend every minute possible devouring whole sets of books from the library bookcase in the back of the classroom; slowly, ruminatingly, but devouring. There was no way my reading could be rushed. Deep twinges of anguish accompanied speed reading drills. I would pretend to be reading faster than I could because I didn't want to be the last student to raise his hand to indicate being finished. Most of all I hated reading tests. If I didn't rush through tests much faster than I could possibly comprehend the material, I would find myself far from the end of the test when the time was called. Yet there were times when I spent all the time I could reading. Books were the entry way to the larger world. The ideas in books were marvelous even if my reading mechanics were tortuous. The ideas in books came to be an important focus of my life, and I would learn to put up with the difficulty for the sake of learning.

Crude drawing was something I did through my childhood, even though I don't remember ever having an art class or being encouraged in any way. In the early grades I would draw what I thought of as the structures of buildings; the beam patterns of skyscrapers and things like that. I was sort of embarrassed for doing these sketches because I didn't know why I wanted to. . . . I just did. Later I took up making crude architectural plans for buildings. I enjoyed music, sang in the chorus, and played different instruments in the band. Music was in me, and if I weren't so shy, I might have been a good musical performer, although I never learned to read music very well.

When I entered algebra class in the ninth grade, the long depression of elementary school ended. Algebra was fascinating to me from the moment I encountered it. In algebra I was the best in my class, and it wasn't just a momentary triumph like when I drew the most accurate length of a yard stick in second grade. My triumph in algebra stuck. In geometry and physics, I was even better. For the physics class in eleventh grade my school was participating in a statewide experiment to see whether instruction through a set of movies was better than regular instruction. My school had regular instruction and my teacher, Mr. Kasle, was good. As a part of the experiment, every other week we would take a special test, which would be sent to a university for scoring. When the scores came back, I would be several points above anyone else in the class. Having lived through the nightmare of the elementary school, I savored every moment of these victories, but savored them in trepidation that they were somehow a fluke, in fear that my incompetencies would descend upon me and I would once again fail. I live in fear of that to this day. It is not easy to free oneself of eight years of degradation when it is experienced at an age too young to have had a chance to know that success is also possible.

Sometime in the ninth grade my class was given a nonverbal IQ test. I don't know exactly how I scored on this test, but there were hints that I had done very well, and after the testing, I was accorded much more respect by my school teachers than before. Had the IQ test been a verbal one, the results, of course, would have been entirely opposite and I would have been seen as anything but brilliant.

There was no program for gifted children in the high school, but the teachers seemed to sense my need and arranged for me to take a correspondence course in advanced algebra. I received a text book in the mail along with my first assignment. I would do my assignments, send them off to the university, and receive them back corrected along with the next assignment. This solitary exercise in doing lists of algebra problems for a disembodied tutor did little to spark my imagination. Though I appreciate the good intention on my behalf in making this arrangement, I would most likely have been better off spending some extra time with Mr. Kasle, the local science teacher who seemed to have a good scientific mind.

The discrepancies in my abilities have persisted. When I took the Graduate Record Exams (GRE) at the completion of undergraduate school, my mathematics score was in the top 2 percent, while my verbal score was just barely in the top quarter. This difference has continually resulted in what to others may seem like an uneven performance. To the extent that tasks depend on a careful understanding of the spatial-mechanical world around me, I usually do quite well. To the extent that it depends on quick verbal analysis, my performance can seem debilitated.

As a child I thought of my problem as personal, and I endured it in silence. Now I cannot be so generous. I see no reason that children who have considerable ability of a distinct kind should be taught that they are inadequate, if not stupid.

A VIEW OF THE SPATIAL CHILD

There are many children who are very capable in their spatial and mechanical understanding of the world around them and at the same time markedly deficient in their efforts to learn reading and writing. Because of their distinct, specialized capabilities, I choose to call them *spatial children*. Spatial children are not prepared to deal with the expectations of school in a conventional way. They often have many difficulties in the early grades of school and spend years being miserably unhappy with their school experience in spite of possessing the capacity for significant accomplishment in life. Yet, most schools remain unprepared to recognize, understand, or serve spatial children. This situation persists even though there has been an accumulation of research information over the past century that can, and should, form the foundation for appropriate work with these children. The information provides a basis for school programming that will allow spatial children to become successful and happy participants in schools.

Spatial ability is not a simple matter. It is not just a picture-like memory for objects, places, and people. This kind of memory might be helpful in carrying out spatial tasks, but it is not at the core of what is meant by spatial ability. Spatial-mechanical thinking involves the capacity to put the world together inside one's head such that all things relate to all others in precisely understood ways. The distance and directional positioning between a whole host of things is so well understood that all become part of an interconnected system. When a person walks through a complex building, it is spatial ability that allows the person to go from one location in the building to another without becoming confused about positioning in relation to all other significant places in the building. This requires a continual readjustment in orientation. Such readjustments may appear to be so instantaneous and automatic that it is wrongly considered a simple, unimportant matter. But psychologists have found that this capacity seems like a simple matter only because it is an aspect of our mental life that we seldom talk about with any precision; unless, of course, we are architects or sculptors and intimate knowledge of the complexities is part of our work. Since we are unable to speak about what is happening in our spatial minds with any precision, we have little appreciation of it. The renowned psychologist, Jean Piaget, has done extensive studies of the development of spatial ability in children. He has found that, when fully developed, spatial ability involves the establishment of an infinite system of interconnected perspectives in a person's mind such that the person can use this system to precisely and simultaneously understand the relationships between a host of things in the physical world.[1] Psychologists and neurologists are most appreciative of spatial ability when patients have completely lost it due to brain damage; such persons may get lost in their own homes or may be unable to dress themselves.

Some would like to think of spatial understanding as if it arrived in a person's head by some act of magic. Spatial ability is not magical. A person arrives at spatial understanding through a long process of mental growth and experience. It may seem intuitive because in some ways it defies verbal analysis. Consider the situation if a law was passed which forbid architects from using blueprints in their work. Describing the plans for a building would take a volume of verbalizations, and still this volume would not do the job as well as a few good blueprints. Because spatial tasks in their gestalt sense defy being carried out in words, those who lack some kind of training in spatial skills have little basis for appreciating its importance or even for recognizing when it is unusually present in a child.

The importance of focusing on spatial ability as a distinct skill is clearly indicated by the problems that have plagued school children when we have failed to do so. Young children whose most distinguished capacities are in spatial tasks often do poorly in school. They have no more basis for understanding their own strengths than do the school teachers who instruct them. These children develop inferiority feelings, which often remain with them for life, in spite of significant adult accomplishments. Sometimes they develop an outright hatred for schools. The child comes to approach all school experience with emotion-laden feelings. This causes severe interference with focusing on the tasks at hand. There may be those few rare moments in the school experience when an art project or a construction project of some kind may catch the child's imagination and keep the child's energies intently focused for a delightful, but brief, interruption of schooling. But then there is the ever-present "necessity" of getting back to the "real" work of school. The child learns that the things that interest him are the rare exceptions in this seemingly endless process called school. Failure to understand the child's unique capacities at times results in very poor guidance of the child. A child who might make a perfectly happy engineer, architect, or mechanic never has exposure to those situations where this kind of work is emphasized or where there are successful role models to emulate. Guidance counselors do not always look for special skill patterns in children and therefore never arrange opportunities for a child to find these things out. If a child with superior spatial ability finds his way into a career in which this ability can be of maximum benefit, it is often more a matter of the child's own good sense and luck than a matter of school personnel understanding and planning for the child's needs. More than a few of the spatial geniuses of history have suffered some variation of this experience before finding an appropriate way of achieving in the world.

THREE CONVERGING LINES OF RESEARCH

Three major lines of psychological research have converged in this century to provide the possibility of a rather clear understanding of the spatial child. These three are (1) studies involving the development of different kinds of tests and use of these tests for predicting career success, (2) studies on learning-disabled and dyslexic children, and (3) research on cerebral asymmetry (on the distinct abilities of the left and right hemispheres of the human brain). The first line of research on various kinds of tests and on prediction of career success was a major focus of interest for psychologists in the first half of this century. Studies indicated that it was of some value to look at tests that emphasized verbal skills and tests that emphasized spatial skills as being rather distinct. A high score on one type of test was often a good indication of possible success in some areas and a high score on the other kind of test was more indicative of success in other areas. For example Frank Holliday, a trainer of engineers in England during the 1930s, did a study in which he used spatial test scores and verbal test scores to predict success in engineering.[2] High scores on spatial tests were found to be good predictors of success in engineering, whereas high scores on verbal tests were much more limited in predicting success in engineering. A few years later, Karl Holzinger and Frances Swineford at the University of Minnesota reported a study involving high school students in which high spatial test scores were predictive of success in science, geometry, and mechanical subjects, but the high spatial test scores were not related whatsoever to exceptional achievement in English and foreign languages.[3] I will review this information further in Chapter 2.

It isn't that verbal test scores and spatial test scores are totally unrelated to each other. Psychologists have found indications that there are aspects of our mental processes that cause all types of abilities to be at about the same level in a given individual. This tendency for all abilities to go together is called *g*, referring to general intelligence. Today psychologists might speculate that this *g* is a reflection of the accuracy with which signals are passed from one neuron to another in the brain. This accuracy allows complex and clearly differentiated mental operations to take place rather than blurred, undifferentiated operations.[4] However, in addition to this *g*, psychologists have found indications that other mental processes don't always go together so well. This is especially true of verbal ability and spatial ability. When verbal ability and spatial ability are separated from *g* through a complex process called *factor analysis,* they are found to be somewhat independent of each other.

This line of research has been most thoroughly reviewed by the English psychologist I. MacFarlane Smith in his book *Spatial Ability: Its Educational and Social Significance.*[5] These findings on relationships between test scores correspond quite well with biographical observations on men of genius. Many people who have been noted for scientific and artistic creativity of a spatial nature have also had difficulty in relating verbally to the social world around them. Sometimes they also had difficulty as children learning to do reading, writing, and arithmetic. This research on the relationship between test scores will be reviewed in more detail in Chapter 3.

The second line of research, that on learning-disabled children, was initiated in the 1920s and 1930s, but was more actively pursued after World War II. Learning-disabled children were sometimes described as having *specific language disability* or *dyslexia*. In other words, the disabilities of many of these children were found to be rather specific to language learning, and there were no neurological signs of any general mental retardation. They could be quite brilliant at constructing things, but when they entered school, they were often at a complete loss in learning to read and write. Sometimes they also had severe difficulties in understanding directions or speaking clearly. Even after these skills were acquired with some difficulty, spelling problems were found to be rampant and persistent. Although psychologists have grown to expect these children, in the early days of the learning-disabilities movement, they were sort of a mystery. There was just no explanation for why children could be capable in many practical skills and at the same time be so disabled in language skills. Some proposed that the children were "word blind." Much of the pioneering work on learning disabilities was stimulated by Doctor Samuel T. Orton, a neurologist who organized a traveling clinic to work with children in rural Iowa during the 1920s.

Long-term study of learning-disabled children led to the observation that whatever the severity of their disability in elementary school, many overcame their difficulties to become accomplished people later in life. Margaret Rawson, a school psychologist following in the Orton tradition, carried out an intensive study of fifty-six boys who had attended a small private school in Pennsylvania. During their childhood, many of the boys had been diagnosed as either moderately or severely disabled in language learning. At the time of the study, these "boys" were adults ranging in age from twenty-six to forty. Rawson was able to compare the adult accomplishments of the boys with the degree of their language disability. In looking at the number of years of higher education achieved, she found that the most disabled group had an average of 6.02 years, the moderately disabled group had 5.69 years, and the nondisabled group had 5.45 years.[6] This is exactly opposite from what one might expect. Rawson also found that the adult job status of the boys followed the same pattern. The most disabled boys had the highest status, the moderately disabled group was next, and the nondisabled group was lowest. Among the twenty most disabled boys, she found two medical doctors, one lawyer, two college professors, two research scientists, three self-employed businessmen, three middle managers, a school principal, three school teachers, and an actor.

Rawson was looking for evidence of the potential of dyslexic boys, but this result surprised her. The boys had obviously conquered many of their problems. To some extent their disability was a developmental lag, which they overcame. However, in other respects, minor language-use problems remained a part of the adult personality of the boys. The lawyer in the group, having succeeded at a rather verbal occupation, indicated that he still wished he could read faster. When asked to explain his success, he said, "The law is based on reason, and so I generally come out with the right answers."[7] The elementary school that these boys attended had a special approach to dyslexic children. Part of this approach was a patient acceptance of the capabilities of a child at any given time. If the child started reading in the second grade rather than the first, this was accepted as the child's own pace of development. This patience may have had a great deal to do with the adjustment of the children in later life.

Perhaps the biggest push to emphasize the skill strengths of learning-disabled children came from Alexander Bannatyne, a psychologist who runs a clinic in Florida.[8] Bannatyne noted that many learning-disabled children are at least average, if not superior, when they are tested on spatial-mechanical activities. He suggested that the brains of these children are organized to be "spatially competent" and that this interferes with language development. Emphasizing the fact that this pattern seems to be an intrinsic part of the child, something they are born with, something that can often be found in their parents and grandparents, Bannatyne chose to call the pattern "genetic dyslexia." More recently, two other clinicians who work with learning-disabled children have identified the same complex of strengths and weaknesses and have chosen to call these children "alpha children."[9] In my own consideration of these children, I would prefer to call them "spatially specialized" or "spatial children." Placing emphasis on a child's strengths and using strengths as a means to eliminate weaknesses is the most important means to raise a child's self-confidence and motivation to learn. We tend to forget this principle too quickly under the pressure of proving our effectiveness as teachers of basic skills. The term *spatial child* will help us to keep this principle in mind.

The third line of research that sheds light on the spatial child comes from observations on cerebral asymmetry. Over the past ten years, it has become popular to talk of being "left-brained" or "right-brained." I want to avoid superficialities in considerations of the research on cerebral asymmetry. However, this research certainly has implications for understanding of the spatial child. For over a century, neurologists have been aware, in some vague sense, that the left hemisphere of our brains is specialized for language and the right hemisphere for visual-spatial processes. Damage to very specific areas of the brain caused by tumors, war injuries, and other unfortunate happenings led to this conclusion. It was seen that when there was injury to one specific part of a person's left hemisphere, he couldn't understand speech. If there was injury to the right hemisphere, the person might get lost trying to find the bathroom in his own house.

The most spectacular blossoming of research and writing on

cerebral asymmetry occurred after a group of neurosurgeons in California severed the neurological connections between the two hemispheres in a group of patients. This surgical procedure relieves the seizures of severely debilitated epileptic patients. It allowed Roger Sperry, the inventor of the procedure, and others, to study the abilities of the two hemispheres with dramatic clarity. After putting together many kinds of observations, a distinct pattern emerged.[10] The left hemisphere has a specialization for detailed, sequential, verbal information. A person tunes in on language and other symbolic processes, and even on the more detailed aspects of graphic information through the left hemisphere. The right hemisphere is specialized for grasping the general, structural relationships in whole objects, spaces, and other systems. It grasps the interconnected complexities of whole systems of information, even perhaps, in things thought to be so unlike as a building and a music composition. This is akin to Jean Piaget's idea of an infinite system of interconnected perspectives by which the world hangs together in one's head. It is just more broadly applied to synthesizing a variety of information in addition to spatial relationships. In 1948, El Koussy speculated that a type of spatial ability was required in music composition.[11] The research of Sperry and others has, perhaps, proven him prophetic.

In trying to make sense of their research, Roger Sperry and Jerre Levy have suggested that the special character of the left hemisphere could be described as "sequential information processing" and the character of the right hemisphere "simultaneous information processing."[12] They have suggested that the two types of processing may be inherently incompatible in the way they are processed by the neurons in our brains. Sequential processing requires a more specialized, predetermined use of certain brain locations. Simultaneous processing requires a more diffuse organization by which larger amounts of information can be "hung together" all at once. This being the case, evolutionary selection has favored a biological separation between the two processes.

The machinery of cerebral asymmetry research is too technically involved to be of much direct use to teachers. It is dominated by corpus callosum surgery, tachistoscopes, electroencephalograms, and Wada tests. This technology is required by researchers as a means of separating the distinct functioning of the two hemispheres. In normal people, the functioning of the two hemispheres is carefully integrated. Information passes from one hemisphere to the other so fast that it is nearly impossible to sort out what is happening where or to make any practical sense of it after we have done so. To the extent that we take on the machinery of the scientist in our work with children, research rather than education tends to become the point of our effort. However, cerebral asymmetry research has two important contributions for educators. First, it provides a dramatic support for the knowledge which educators already had, i.e. that verbal ability and spatial ability are of a rather distinct, separate nature and that in some sense they may be incompatible. The idea of their separateness becomes neurologically based. The fact that there are some people in whom spatial-type skills predominate and other people in whom verbal-type skills predominate becomes very reasonable. The other value of cerebral asymmetry research is that it points educators toward making other kinds of observations that were already hinted at by previous research. Among spatial children, educators can be sensitive to watching for a special approach to music, a special approach to creativity, a special approach to literature and poetry, and a special emotional tone. I will return to the research on cerebral asymmetry in Chapter 5.

I have been briefly reviewing three lines of research on psychological testing, learning-disabled children, and cerebral asymmetry. These have converged in a dramatic way during this century to provide a solid foundation for teachers to understand one type of difference between children. It is essential that school teachers have at least some familiarity with this research and with its implications for their work.

BIOGRAPHY

In studying children who are rather specialized for spatial thinking, it is valuable to look at biographical information. Psychological research, like that reviewed in the section above, gives a very general, disembodied view of people. These generalities allow an educator to assert with confidence that the research has implications for a broad spectrum of children. Biographical study, on the other hand, allows us a greater feeling of "realness" about our concerns.

Since I am working from the perspective of education for gifted children, I find it most interesting to look at the lives of people who have become famous for their spatial genius. Among these people there are many who are obvious candidates for being considered spatial children. In other words, there is evidence that they had language learning difficulties as children, but distinguished themselves as spatial thinkers. Pablo Picasso, Albert Einstein, the French sculptor Auguste Rodin, the outstanding American surgeon Harvey Cushing, Isaac Newton, Leonardo DaVinci, the German founder of chemotherapy Paul Ehrlich, Niels Bohr, and Thomas Alva Edison have all been described in this way by those in the learning disabilities movement. In Chapter 4, I will go into detailed case studies of Albert Einstein and Pablo Picasso. In this section, I would like briefly to introduce biography with the case of Isaac Newton, the preeminent genius of the seventeenth century, the describer of the workings of gravity, the inventor of calculus, and the mathematical formulator of the pathways of moons, planets, and stars. For nearly three centuries, until another spatial child by the name of Albert Einstein came along, Newton's thinking dominated the field of physics.

Isaac Newton was born in 1642 in the small farming hamlet of Woolsthorpe in central England. There was nothing in his family background that might suggest the foundation for genius. His father was a relatively prosperous lord of the manor. He was described as a "wild, extravagant, and weak man"; he certainly was no scholar or scientist.[13] His mother was an intelligent, prudent woman who provided much love and support for Newton, but nothing in her character suggests unusual creativity. Newton grew up in disturbing and unsettled circumstances. His father died two months before his birth. That same year the English Civil War broke out; its most violent activities took place in the vicinity of Woolsthorpe. The prosperity of his family allowed that even under these conditions, he was able to attend school, first at two local day schools and then from age twelve to age nineteen at the Kings School in Grantham, a larger community nearby.

Detailed records on the school achievement of a country boy growing up in the middle of the seventeenth century is more than historians could hope for. From the information available, however, one thing is certain. In the early years of school, Newton was a most unimpressive student. When he entered Grantham School, he was placed in the "lowest form" and at one point he was "last in the lower-most class but one"; i.e. there was perhaps only one boy in the school who was performing in a more disappointing manner than poor Isaac.[14] Years later, after Isaac Newton had established himself as an unchallenged genius, a national hero, and a mental celebrity of the proportions that Einstein was in this century, a group of his classmates collaborated in writing a statement of memories about their most famous fellow student. At the time, Newton's legend was being used as an example of the genius of the English people and the former classmates were undoubtedly under the expectation of having the most glowing memories of Isaac. Nonetheless, they had to report in all honesty that "dull boys were now and then put over him in form."

One might ask in what kinds of school work was Newton doing so poorly when he entered Grantham School. There is no certain way to answer this question. No detailed evaluation of his school work is available. We can, however, make some fairly certain guesses at the problem by considering the nature of the standard curriculum at the school. In addition to the usual emphasis in elementary schools on reading, writing, and arithmetic, when Newton began his preparation for the university, there was a very strong emphasis on the classical languages: Latin, Greek, and probably Hebrew. During the seventeenth century, these languages were still the medium of common intellectual discourse in the universities of Europe. Attendance at Cambridge University would have been impossible had Newton not been well prepared in these languages. In addition to this emphasis on language, some instruction was given in ancient history and theology. In mathematics, his instruction went little beyond the computational basics of arithmetic. Since Newton was known to have a special appreciation for ancient history and was known to readily use mathematics computation in his own creative work as a child, it is quite certain that his academic difficulties were primarily with languages.[15] His academic prospects were evidently considered to be so limited that after Newton completed four years of study at Grantham School, his mother decided that it would be better for him to stay at home and learn to manage the farm. Newton's stepfather had recently died, and it was decided that if Newton didn't have much future in an intellectual career, he should just as well prepare to take over the family farm.[16]

The other side of this story is that at the same time Newton was being placed in the lowest form, next to the lowest in his class, and beneath dull boys, everyone was seeing the ingenious side of his personality. In their description, his former classmates reported that he was continually engaged in mechanical experiments.

> He always busied himself in making knick-knacks and models of wood in many kinds. For which purpose he had got little saws, hatchets, hammers, and all sorts of tools, which he would use with great dexterity. . . . All holidays, and what time the boys had allowed to play, he spent entirely in knocking and hammering in his lodging room, pursuing that strong bent of his inclination not only in things serious, but ludicrous too, and what would please his school-fellows, as well as himself.[17]

He was reported to have made a wooden clock, a model of a local windmill, and special kites. His windmill was built to house a mouse and was so cleverly constructed that the mouse's efforts to receive corn from the mill caused the mill to turn. The workings of the mill were somewhat of a mystery and a point of conjecture by the other students.

Two circumstances resulted in Newton not spending the rest of his life as a farmer. First, there were influential adults who recognized his special genius, and second, his mother found that he was obviously not very well suited to be a good farmer. One of Newton's guardian angels was the headmaster of Grantham School, a Mr. Stokes. The other was Mr. Clark, an apothecary. Mr. Clark was a friend of the Newton family, and Newton lodged with the Clarks while at Grantham School. While the Headmaster Mr. Stokes may have been frustrated by Newton's slowness in scholarly skills, he evidently saw the other side of genius, and he encouraged Newton's mother to allow the boy to return to Grantham School. For his part, Mr. Clark, the apothecary, had been encouraging Newton's mechanical investigations, introduced Newton to an interest in chemistry, and had backed up Mr. Stokes' insistence that the boy should return to school. In the meantime, "farmer Isaac" was spending much of his time being absentmindedly preoccupied with his thoughts — losing his horse while walking up a hill absorbed in reading and avoiding his lessons in farm bartering in order to sneak away to Mr. Clark's house to continue his investigations. There was no use in insisting that he become a farmer, and he returned to Grantham School to finish his preparation for Cambridge University.

We should look briefly at Newton's character because it gives us a clear and rather typical example of the personality of the spatial child. Miss Storey, who was Mr. Clark's stepdaughter, and Newton's closest childhood playmate and fiancée for many years before Newton decided to remain an academically engrossed bachelor, was once asked to describe his character. She remembered him as a quiet, introspective boy who enjoyed playing with her girlfriends: "Sir Isaac was always a sober, silent, thinking lad, and was never known scarce to play with the boys abroad, at their silly amusements; but would rather choose to be at home, even among the girls, and would frequently make little tables, cupboards, and other utensils for her and her playfellows, to set their babies and trinkets on."[18]

Most interesting in this description is the "sober, silent, thinking lad," suggestive of the introverted, social aloofness that considerable research has come to associate with distinctive spatial ability. It was said that he "jealously and persistently guarded the sanctuary of his mind" and that "he was cold and formal, and was singularly unable to form intimate friendships."[19] As a student at Cambridge, he tended to be socially ignored by both the rowdier types and the more studious types; by the former because he "shunned all forms of physical exercise, played no games, and disliked boys" and by the latter because he "was not sociable, witty, or talkative by nature."[20] The asocial nature of his character occasionally was such that he would become suspicious that other people were attempting to rob him of his ideas. He would become involved in petty disputes.

Another salient part of his character was an interest in art and poetry. As an adult, Newton disdained taking the arts seriously at all, but nevertheless, as a boy, he dabbled in the arts considerably. When he stayed at Mr. Clark's house, the whole wall of his room was filled with drawings of "birds, beasts, men, ships and mathematical schemes."[21] Newton wrote some verse, and one of his poems has survived. It is about King Charles I. In the English Civil War, Newton's family sided with the Royalists, and the young Newton was an admirer of King Charles I, who was executed when Isaac was seven years old.[22] The latent interest in the arts, which Newton evidently repressed as an adult, is meaningful to those with an interest in cerebral asymmetry research. Some of this research suggests that the right hemisphere, in addition to playing a special part in spatial ability, provides a foundation for creative expression. If a child has special precocity for spatial ability, might it be appropriate to look for an accompanying inclination toward creative expression? Some learning-disabilities clinicians think this connection is common.

One of the more interesting items from Newton's life is a little 2¾-inch-by-4⅞-inch notebook that he kept as a boy. This notebook was missing for nearly a century and then showed up in the Pierpont Morgan Library in the 1920s. In the part of the notebook dating from his studies at Grantham School is the description of a system Newton invented for phonetic writing. In the part of the book dating from the time he was a student at Cambridge, there is a plan for the reform of spelling.[23] The fact that one of the most creative scientists in history would spend time trying to reform writing and spelling is intriguing. The English language has an almost total lack of phonetic consistency. This is the source of some of the most prevalent difficulties for spatial children. The lack of consistency turns all pronunciation and spelling into a mammoth memorization task, most disconcerting for those having an orderly mind. Perhaps in his attempt to find a solution to the problem, the youthful Newton was revealing to history the source of some of his own difficulties in school. He was certainly three centuries ahead of current attempts to introduce phonetic consistency into the English language, such as the initial alphabet and words in color. I will deal with this problem in more detail in Chapter 10.

Isaac Newton was a lucky spatial child. In spite of his initial difficulties in school, several influential adults seemed to have an intuitive sense of his unique capacities; they encouraged him to continue working toward an academic career. It is to their credit that he arrived in the world of ideas where he could make his gargantuan contribution to understanding of the physical world. Very often, when spatial children do survive the problems of early school with their self-confidence intact, it can be seen that the help and support of one or more influential adults was crucial to their having done so.

It would not be appropriate to attempt to generalize from case studies on geniuses like Newton to every child in learning-disabilities classrooms. Newton is, to say the least, an unusual case. Few people in history have the creative capacity to accomplish what he did. It would be as big a mistake to expect learning-disabled children to turn into Isaac Newtons as it would be to overlook potential for above average accomplishment among many learning-disabled children. However, case studies like this suggest confidence in the more generalizable research by pointing out correspondences, e.g. interests of the spatial child in creative expression and tendencies for the spatial child to have a rather introverted personality.

A SOCIAL CONFLICT IN THE CLASSROOM THEORY

Carl Sagan, the astronomer and writer, has given an interesting view of research on cerebral asymmetry. In his book, *The Dragons of Eden*, Sagan suggests that conflict between global, intuitive thinkers and verbal, analytic thinkers runs throughout human history, i.e. between right-hemisphere thinking and left-hemisphere thinking.[24] He suggests that it would be better if such a conflict was not a pervasive part of our mental lives.

As Sagan sees it, the conflict has usually taken place on a subtle, subterranean level, since the case for the right hemisphere is seldom represented in verbal form; that is not the effective mode of the right hemisphere. It is a struggle in which the verbal mode has been in the ascendancy throughout civilized history — dependent as civilized man is on endless verbal transactions. However, on occasion, the ascendancy surfaces in not so subtle ways, such as when in many traditional cultures, the left hand (controlled by and expressive of the right hemisphere) was reserved for toilet wiping duties and it was considered offensive to use the left hand in any other way such as in shaking hands or eating; when the right side of the king or God was designated as the place of honor, and the left side the place of disgrace; or when the word *left* became linguistically equated with all that is vile, sinister, weak, worthless, awkward, and deceitful, and the word *right* became associated in various languages with propriety, grace, and rectitude.[25] Such a consistency could only derive from a motivation that is seriously compelling even if not consciously recognized. It perhaps derives from a defensive insecurity among verbal thinkers that their position may somehow be in doubt, from a need to use irrationalities to justify the common social domination by the verbally astute. Sagan suggests that the most distinctive achievements of man have derived from a cooperative mentality in which global intuitions and symbolic analyses are brought to bear at the same time on the same problems. In this, Sagan is undoubtedly correct. However, this kind of cooperative mentality can hardly be consistantly achieved until equal social importance is assigned to global, intuitive thinking and until those who are most capable of global, intuitive thinking are given better opportunities to make their proper contribution.

It is very likely that the struggles of spatial children to survive in school are lonely, dispersed, micro-level parts of the larger social, historical conflict of which Sagan speaks. More than anything else, on the larger social scale, elementary school represents the efforts of a society to quickly and efficiently introduce young children into the standard, official, symbolic modes of the society in which they will be adult participants. Elementary school teachers are often those who themselves experienced comfort and success when they were being introduced in first grade to the memorized intricacies of reading, writing, and arithmetic. Training for elementary school teaching appropriately has a strong emphasis on these basic subjects. Some teachers are prepared to teach science and to use manipulative materials for teaching mathematics. However, it is the rare teacher who has any extensive training in the nature of spatial and mechanical skills or who uses spatially dominant activities as anything but a passing fancy in the classroom. This being the case, teachers are rarely in a position to draw either on their own experiences as children or on their professional training to provide a basis for understanding the spatial child.

There are school children who have the potential for understanding the interconnected patterns in quantum theory, quasars, path analysis, thermodynamics, matrix algebra, spatial analysis, etc. For this they need a receptive sensitivity to the interconnected complexities of the world around them, a complexly organized mind, a capacity for seeing how the global view and the analytic view of the world can fit together. Some of these same children have trouble deciphering *Dick and Jane* in the first grade. At the very least, schools should be expected to set up arrangements through which these children can be discovered and provided for.

Albert Einstein, a spatial child of the first order, once gave his impression of his own school experience. Einstein as a child was so slow in language development that his parents feared he might be subnormal. Yet, he was so obviously gifted in the complexity of his thoughts that a scientifically inclined friend of the Einstein family voluntarily undertook his tutoring in some of the more advanced ideas of science and philosophy. I will present more of the biographic details on Einstein in Chapter 4. At this point, let me quote from his impression of his own school experience given at an address at the State University of New York: "The teachers in the elementary school appeared to me like sergeants and in the Gymnasium (high school) the teachers were like lieutenants. . . . The worst thing seems to be for a school principally to work with methods of fear, force, and artificial authority. Such treatment destroys the healthy feelings, the integrity, and self-confidence of the pupils. All that it produces is a servile helot."[26] For a kindly soul like Albert Einstein to make such a bitter statement is quite amazing. For him to make this statement after he had clearly established himself among the geniuses of all time, this is doubly amazing. A close look at the biographical evidence suggests that this bitterness was surfacing from the deeper levels of frustration and anger of a spatial child who had flunked out of school in spite of his brilliance.

Too many highly gifted children have suffered misery and alienation in the school experience (Picasso, Einstein, Edison, Rodin, Newton, and Churchill, to name a few). It might be hoped that at some point in our efforts to understand the intricacies of the educational process, we would learn how to avoid alienating some of the most brilliant children who pass under our care. It would be a grand landmark achievement. If we are to do so then, our understanding must go beyond the simplistic and repetitious intonation that we do in fact alienate many brilliant children. We must understand why we do. Part of that landmark achievement will lay in our studied understanding of the spatial child. Considering the contributions that spatial children have made to the world, we owe it to them to make the attempt.

REFERENCES

1. Piaget, J., and Inhelder, B. *The Child's Concept of Space*. New York: Norton and Co., 1967.
2. Holliday, F. A study into the selection of apprentices for the engineering industry. *Occupational Psychology, 14*:69-81, 1940.
3. Holzinger, K.J., and Swineford, F. The relation of two bi-factors to achievement in geometry and other subjects. *The Journal of Educational Psychology,*

37:261-265, 1946.

4. Eysenck, H.J. Brain wave measurements confirm I.Q. test results. *Bulletin of the Leadership Training Institute, 7*:3, 1980.

5. Smith, I.M. *Spatial Ability: Its Educational and Social Significance.* London: University of London Press, 1964.

6. Rawson, M. *Developmental Language Disability: Adult Accomplishments of Dyslexic Boys.* Baltimore: Johns Hopkins Press, 1968.

7. *Ibid.,* p. 55.

8. Bannatyne, A. *Language, Reading and Learning Disabilities.* Springfield, Ill.: Charles C Thomas, Publisher, 1971.

9. Fadely, J., and Hosler, V. *Understanding the Alpha Child at Home and School.* Springfield, Ill.: Charles C Thomas, Publisher, 1979.

10. Levy-Agresti, J., and Sperry, R. Differential perceptual capacities in major and minor hemispheres. *Proceedings of the National Academy of Sciences, 61*:1151, 1968.

11. Smith, *op. cit.,* p. 211.

12. Levy-Agresti and Sperry, *op. cit.,* p. 1151.

13. More, L. *Isaac Newton.* New York: Charles Scribner's Sons, 1935, p. 3.

14. *Ibid.,* p. 11.

15. *Ibid.,* p. 9.

16. *Ibid.,* p. 6.

17. *Ibid.,* pp. 12-13.

18. *Ibid.,* p. 16.

19. *Ibid.,* pp. 14-17.

20. *Ibid.,* p. 42.

21. *Ibid.,* p. 14.

22. *Ibid.,* p. 15.

23. *Ibid.,* pp. 18-19.

24. Sagan, C. *The Dragons of Eden.* New York: Random House, 1977.

25. *Ibid.,* pp. 155-158.

26. Kuznetsov, B. *Einstein.* Moscow: 1965, p. 22.

Chapter 2

WHAT IS SPATIAL ABILITY?

A T face value, spatial ability seems as if it should be fairly straightforward and simple. After all, it deals with the objects and the spaces between objects in the world around us. We have been looking at that world, and touching and feeling it, from the time we were born. We have learned to deal with that space quite well. We can find our way around in it. We recognize most of the things we encounter, and we quickly become accustomed to new objects. How could the fact that some children emphasize spatial perceptions and spatial understanding be of any important consequence? In order to be able to answer this question, it is important to recognize that spatial ability is not a simple matter. Children do not reach their full potential in spatial reasoning until after puberty, until they have had more than ten years of exploring in the world. I will return to Jean Piaget's description of this lengthy developmental process later in this chapter.

It is important to make a distinction between the gross, perceptual recognition of shapes or objects and the understanding of spatial relationships within these shapes or objects. In order to make this distinction clear, those readers who are not trained artists should try the following exercise. Take a blank piece of paper and draw the face of your best friend. Try it! Would another person recognize this as a drawing of the face of your friend? Perhaps they would, and perhaps they wouldn't. You know the face of your friend as a whole perceptual entity so well that you would never, ever mistake your friend for anyone else. Yet your attempt to draw your friend may be completely dissatisfying to you. Part of your difficulty may be in getting proper control over your hand so that it will do what you want it to do on an unfamiliar task. Most likely, the larger part of your difficulty is a lack of knowledge of the relationships and patterns in the face being drawn. How are the eyes positioned in relation to the bridge of the nose? What is the proper outline of the face going from the cheek bones to the chin? What are the usual kinds of shading patterns in a face? How do all of these things change when the face is seen from different angles? These may have been some of the questions going through your mind as you were drawing your friend's face. Your unfailing knowledge of your friend's face as a whole perceptual entity may be in complete contrast to your lack of knowledge of the specific relationships that make up that whole perceptual entity. This is probably like the experience of a young child who has learned to recognize, and even name, a square, and yet is unable to draw a square accurately. Lack of knowledge of relationships in the square (straightness of lines, perpendicularity of angles, parallelism of sides) undermines the effort.

What then is spatial ability? Spatial understanding depends on grasping the consistency in relationships between things when these relationships occur in the context of fluid, changing patterns. The fluidity presents infinite possibilities like a face seen from different angles. But the grasp of the relationships holds this infinity together to accomplish two things. First, grasp of the relationships allows people to recognize that they are seeing different instances of the same thing within the fluid, infinite possibilities of the pattern, because the relationships remain consistent. Second, grasp of the relationships allows a person to anticipate instances in the infinite flow of possibilities, even though the person may never actually have observed that given instance before.

All this is abstract; so let's look at an example. Suppose you were shown a block like the top one illustrated in Figure 2-1. You would think it somewhat simple to determine that another observation on a different occasion could be of the same block turned a different way or seen from a different perspective as shown in the middle illustration of Figure 2-1. On the other hand, there are other observations of blocks that would never lead you to say you are seeing the same block, e.g. the bottom illustration in Figure 2-1. The relationships in the dimensions are different; the positioning of the shading has changed.

All three of these drawings look different to your eye, but two of them you see as possibly being the same block. Long periods of playing with the objects of the world when you were a child has taught you that a given thing may look different depending on the position from which you see it; yet it is the same thing. You recognize that spatial relationships in the object are maintained, even when you view these relationships from a different angle. Sensitivity to the preservation of spatial relationships in the object itself, in spite of a

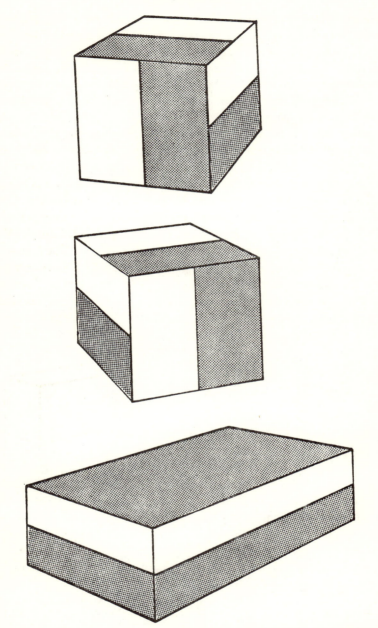

Figure 2-1. Even though the top and middle block designs are physically different as they appear in a flat surface illustration, knowledge of spatial relationships suggests that they might be illustrations of the same block turned in a different direction. Knowledge of spatial relationships suggests that the bottom block design would never be mistaken for the upper two.

changed angle of observation, is crucial to your being able to determine when you are seeing an object that you have seen before. You are sensitive to the maintenance of relationships, in spite of the infinite fluid possibilities within which they may be observed. You are also sensitive to when relationships have not been maintained, and this becomes the clue that you are looking at something different.

In addition to being able to tell when you are seeing the same object, you can also imagine in your mind what an object would look like from a position you have never seen it before. If I asked you to draw one of the blocks in Figure 2-1, but as seen from a different angle of observation, you would be able to do a credible job, even though you have never actually seen the block from the new perspective. You grasp relationships between length, width, and depth. You observe the relationships in the patterns on the blocks. You know, at least roughly, how these relationships are pictorially preserved when the block is placed in different positions. If I asked you to draw the same block in an infinite number of different positions, you could probably begin doing this with satisfaction that you were doing all right.

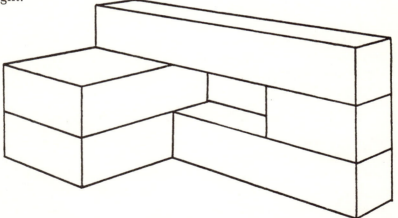

Figure 2-2. Try to imagine this block structure as it might be seen from the opposite side and then draw it.

When the idea of spatial skill is put in terms like this, it might seem rather unimpressive. However, if we move very little beyond the familiar block shape to a more complicated object, the difficulties multiply. Try to imagine a structure like the one in Figure 2-2 from an angle opposite to that shown. Could you draw a credible representation of the structure as it might be seen from the opposite side?

PIAGET'S OBSERVATIONS
ON THE DEVELOPMENT OF SPATIAL ABILITY

Understanding of spatial relationships in even the simple block examples above are much more involved than commonly thought. It involves the integration of a set of skills we hardly knew we had until Jean Piaget brought them into focus through his brilliant studies. Piaget carried out long and extensive observations on the development of spatial skills in children. A full understanding of his work is not easy to attain, and it would be presumptuous to suggest that a full understanding could be offered here. Nevertheless, a brief review of some of his work will help make clear some of the skills that are involved in the most basic spatial abilities. It will also help to make clear the gradual process by which children come to acquire these skills and integrate them so that the skills can be applied to more complex spatial problems.

Jean Piaget has proposed that the full spatial understanding of the child evolves from three different groups of related skills. These are skills involved in understanding *topological relationships,* skills involved in understanding *projective relationships,* and skills involved in understanding *Euclidean relationships.*

Topological Space

Topological relationships involve such things as proximity, separation, order, enclosure, and continuity. These are the simplest of spatial relationships, but the basis for the development of all others. *Proximity* is the observation that two things occur near each other. *Separation* is the observation that although two things may be in close proximity, they are distinct, separate things. *Order* means that a sequence is observed, i.e. three or more separate objects remain in some consistent order. Essential to the full comprehension of order is the ability to reverse order and to see that this reversal represents the same ordered relationship seen from the opposite direction. *Enclosure* is the observation that something is surrounded by other things. *Continuity* is the observation that although a number of objects may be focused on as distinct from each other, they all occur together in certain continuous relationships, so that they make up some whole entity.

When young children first acquire sensitivity to topological relationships, it is within the flowing perceptions of the fluid world that surrounds them. For example these observations might be made about the faces of other people. The nose is in proximity to the mouth. Yet the two have a separateness. The forehead, nose, and mouth occur in a certain ordered relationship, and this order can be seen in one direction or as reversed from another direction. The nose is enclosed by the cheeks. Yet all of these objects form a perceptual continuity that the child comes to recognize as a whole face.

Let's look at one example of the way Piaget studied the development of topological understanding. Piaget continually emphasized the importance of haptic perception — touching, feeling and handling of objects — as necessary for understanding the spatial world. For the child, vision by itself tends to present gross, undifferentiated, two-dimensional patterns. The child can associate these patterns with certain events and thus give them significance. When the mother arrives with bottle in hand, it means the child will get fed. But the child acquires little knowledge of the spatial structure of objects from this perception. It is when the child starts touching and handling the objects around him and begins relating these experiences to what is seen that the child begins to make the most elementary steps toward understanding of spatial structure.

In order to study the way children relate what they see to what they touch and feel, Piaget placed a screen in front of children in such a way that by putting their hands underneath the screen they could handle objects but not see them. Sometimes these might be common objects, such as a pencil, a key, or a comb. Other times these would be cardboard cutouts of common geometric shapes, such as circles, squares, triangles, or crosses. There were also cutouts of irregular shapes — some with holes, some open or closed irregular rings, some intertwined rings.

The children were asked to give different responses depending on the object and the age level of the child. Sometimes they were asked to name an object; sometimes they were asked to choose the object they were handling behind the screen from a set of several drawings of objects that they could see; and sometimes they were asked to draw the object.

Before the age of two and one-half years, children had considerable difficulty participating in this haptic perception activity because they rejected the idea of handling objects they couldn't see, i.e. screens are for looking under. Between age two and one-half and three and one-half, children began successful participation in the activity and they could recognize familiar objects, e.g. a key or pencil. Most could not recognize other shapes that were being handled. Children expressed confidence as they were handling a square and then identified it by pointing to the picture of a circle. Some children would indicate that they could draw pictures of objects but then produced what appeared to be scribbling. They would grasp an object but not explore it from point to point. Without such exploratory behavior, the part of the object that happened to be grasped became the focus in the attempt to identify the object. If the straight side of a triangle was grasped, then the straight side of a square became an acceptable equivalent and the child failed to select the correct figure.

Between ages three and one-half and four, children began to distinguish objects on the basis of some of the grossest topological features, such as enclosure. An open ring was distinguished from a closed ring, because of the large opening on one side. But the child tended not to distinguish between a circle and a square. The exploratory behavior of the child was increasing, but it was still random and unorganized. This random exploration brought attention to larger featural differences, but not to finer details nor to the way these details related to each other.

Around age five, the children Piaget studied began to notice angles and corners. They first noticed these as things that stick out from the smooth surfaces of other parts of objects. As one child put it, "It's something that pricks." The children also began to explore in the two directions from corners and angles to develop the idea that corners are places where lines meet. This helped to distinguish curving lines that don't have distinct pointing angles from objects that consist of sets of straight lines, and therefore do. When this occurred, the children could distinguish circles from squares, but they still had difficulty distinguishing squares from triangles. Without a coordinated exploration of the whole object, the triangle seemed no different from a diamond or square. Drawings began to take on some of the angular features, but they were a reflection of the exploratory behavior, or as Piaget* put it, "drawing expresses the child's exploratory movements rather than his visual perception, even when he afterwards has the models before his eyes."[1] A diamond was sometimes drawn as an oblong figure with a point attached on either end as in Figure 2-3.

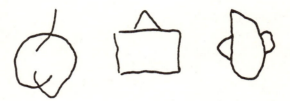

Figure 2-3. Early attempts to draw a diamond when a child discovers that it is an object with points that stick out. From J. Piaget and B. Inhelder, *The Child's Conception of Space,* 1967. Reprinted by permission of Humanities Press Inc., Atlantic Highlands, N.J. 07716 and Routledge & Kegan Paul Ltd., London, England.

As the children approached age six, their exploration became more active. There were more hesitations as they attempted to relate various discovered features to each other. Systematic exploration is not quite achieved. "The child explores everything but keeps moving ahead all the time, never returning systematically to obtain a stable point of reference."[2] The children were able to draw simpler shapes with ease, but they had considerable difficulty with more complex shapes, such as stars.

Around age seven, the exploration of the children began to take on features of what Piaget called operational behavior, i.e. "action which can return to its starting point, and which can be integrated with other actions also possessing this feature of reversibility."[3] This operational behavior allowed the children to use reference points to integrate an object as a whole. By using direction and distance from a reference point to locate a key feature, and then returning to the reference point, the child was prepared to move off in a new direction to find another key feature, which could then be more exactly related to the first in terms of the reference point, the direction, and

---

*From Jean Piaget and Barbel Inhelder, *The Child's Conception of Space,* 1967. Reprinted by permission of Humanities Press Inc., Atlantic Highlands, N.J. 07716 and Routledge & Kegan Paul Ltd., London, England.

the distance. The reversibility in operational behavior thus becomes crucial to the integration of a whole object in a child's mind.

> Tus (7.9 years) draws crosses, half-crosses, etc., correctly. Six-pointed star; explores the six arms, returning systematically to the center to co-ordinate them. He draws it correctly, checking each arm in turn by going back to the central reference point . . . (this results in) grouping the elements perceived in terms of a general plan, and starting from a fixed point of reference to which the child can always return. . . . Every element explored is at the same time distinct, yet connected with all the rest in a single coherent whole.[4]

In describing this sequence of skill development, it should be pointed out that the gross topological features are the first to be discovered. Whether an object was open or closed and the way this was implied by proximity, separateness, and continuity were observed first. More geometric types of relationships, such as the sizes of angles, obviously were beginning to enter into the understanding of the children as they made accurate drawings of squares and diamonds. Nevertheless, it was the topological relationships that first became noticeable in their attempts to distinguish between objects.

Projective Space

A second cluster of spatial skills involve projection along a line of sight. Understanding projection along a line of sight is fundamental to knowing that the position we see something from determines how it appears, i.e. perspective. This cluster of skills starts with a child determining when a number of objects are lined up with each other. The full development of projective skills isn't reached until children can create in their mind a fairly accurate image of how objects or groups of objects would look from any direction or distance, even though they have seen the objects from only one position. This does not involve knowing that there is a polar bear on the other side of the mountain when you have never seen the bear; however it does involve being able to imagine with fair accuracy how the mountain would be positioned in relation to other mountains if you were to look at the mountains from an entirely different direction. In other words, it involves the imagination and coordination in your mind of the infinite possibilities of lines of sight.

Piaget's first step in the study of perspective was to make observations on the way the concept of a straight line develops. Piaget asked children to imagine that match sticks were telephone poles and then asked them to stick these into a plasticine base to form a straight line. The younger children under four years of age could recognize a straight line and pick one out from pictures representing both straight and curved lines; however the same children were quite unable to construct a straight line. They could follow a straight line by placing the match sticks right along the straight edge of a base, but when the line was to be constructed at any distance from the edge, the line would become very wavy and irregular.

Between ages four and seven, the children moved toward constructing a fairly straight line when the straight edge of the base could be used as a guide, even if the line was to be constructed at some distance from the guiding edge. One of the problems at this stage was that if the guiding edge of a base itself was not straight (e.g. if it was circular), the child would still try to follow it in constructing the straight line. If the two points between which the child was to construct a line were not parallel with an edge, the child would be thrown off by trying to use the edge as a guide. The children were attempting to use their sensitivity to straight objects in the world around them as the primary reference for their constructions. When this worked, they succeeded. When it didn't, they failed.

Around age seven, the children developed the appropriate concrete operational strategy. They began to realize that their own line of sight could be used as a means for constructing a straight line, a means that was independent of the objects around them, so that it could not be thrown off by these objects. By placing themselves in a position such that the starting point and the end point are at the same place in their line of sight and then placing match sticks between these points, the children could construct a straight line without reference to any other objects. Awareness of this available concrete operation develops slowly in the child. Piaget would sometimes try to guide younger children toward discovering the line-of-sight method by placing them in the right position for sighting. It generally would do little good. Younger children would be unready to use this concrete operation; they would return to their former methods and to their mistakes.

This study of the child's attempts to construct a straight line and of the child's discovery of the line of sight was Piaget's starting point in understanding skills related to projective space. A fuller development of these skills comes when a child is able to imagine different perspectives on groups of objects and to coordinate these perspectives to accurately anticipate what the objects would look like from a different direction or distance. In order to study this higher level development, Piaget created a pasteboard model of three mountains. One mountain had a small house on it, another had a cross on top, and the tallest mountain was capped by snow. These details were intended to keep the mountains distinctly clear in the child's mind. In addition to the model, Piaget also used large pictures of the model as it would be seen from different directions. He also used a small doll that could be placed in different positions around the model to represent a person seeing the model from these different positions.

Piaget tested for the coordination of perspectives in different ways. Sometimes children were asked to rearrange the separate mountains to reconstruct the way the whole model would be seen from other positions. These other perspectives around the model were represented to the child by placing the doll in different positions facing the model. Another procedure was to have the child pick out the one picture that best represented what the mountains would look like from where the doll was sitting. Piaget would ask the child to "show me what a snapshot of the mountains would look like if it were taken by the doll from where it sees the mountains." In a third procedure, the child was shown a picture and then asked to indicate where the doll would need to sit in order to see that view of the mountains. Let's look at how this coordination of infinite possible perspectives develops in the child.

Children under age four show no indication that they understand the activity at all. These children apparently have no grasp of what it might be like to see things from another person's line of sight without first moving to the other person's viewing position. Children between ages five and seven can place the separate mountains in positions such that they provide an accurate representation of the model as viewed from the child's position. When, however, the child is asked to imagine the view from any other position (as indicated by where the doll is sitting), the child will manipulate the separate mountains as if to represent the model from a different viewpoint, but inevitably position them as they were before; i.e. representing the child's own point of view. Even if the child has had a previous opportunity to see the model from a different position, which the child is now trying to imagine, the child at this stage still tends to give a representation appropriate to his current viewing position. When asked to pick out from a number of pictures the one that best represents the doll's point of view, the child picks out the one representing his own point of view. If given a picture representing a different position from his own and asked to place the doll in a position appropriate to the viewpoint of the picture, the child is virtually lost, often placing the doll in the middle of the mountains in response to all of the pictures. The essential feature of the child's efforts at this point is that "the child considers his present point of view the only possible one . . . he imagines that he sees the entire group of mountains as it really is in some way which is common to any and every perspective."[5]

At age seven or eight, the child begins to make a transition away from this egocentric viewpoint. The attempt to represent the doll's point of view results in various kinds of shifting in the placement of the mountains away from the child's point of view. These shifts, however, generally represent little more than the child's recognition of needing to do something different. The changes seem to be random. Sometimes the child shows a very slight but interesting shift. The child places the mountains in such a way, facing the doll, that the doll can see the mountains the way the child sees them; i.e. the child's viewpoint is still central, and the child is attempting to make it possible for the doll to see the world the way the child sees it, rather than the child attempting to achieve the doll's viewpoint. The child remains tied to a "single false-absolute viewpoint."[6] When the child attempts to choose a picture representing the doll's viewpoint, the one accurate guiding factor that enters at this stage is distance. If the doll is near a particular mountain, the child will choose a picture that has that mountain in the foreground. The child will often make a mistake on left and right positioning, often choosing a left-right positioning that is correct from the child's point of view rather than the doll's.

At age eight or nine, the child begins to accurately shift to the doll's point of view. Left and right relationships are worked out as well as foreground and background relationships. This is gradual, and there is much experimenting as the child proceeds. Relation-

ships tend to be corrected one by one rather than the child taking
thought to determine what the complete final pattern should look
like and reproducing that image as a whole. As children reach age
nine or ten, they begin dealing with the various relationships all
together. The child can achieve a complete mental image of a possible solution and place each mountain, in turn, in such a way that all
of the relationships are considered with each placement. In Piaget's
words, "the reasoning which takes place involves the coordination or
multiplication of relationships."[7]

In order to appreciate the full complexity of what children
achieve at this final stage, it must be realized that they are, in their
mind's eye, coordinating any one perspective with the infinite variety of all other possible perspectives. Children can accurately imagine any of these infinite possible perspectives, even when they have
never actually experienced them before.

> No single perspective, no one visual picture corresponding to a particular
> point of view, can render the spatial character of the group of mountains
> as a whole. This can only be done by means of operations enabling one
> perspective to be linked with the rest. That is to say, by operations that
> link a particular perspective with the universe of possible perspectives. To
> put it another way, the reason why no single perspective can embrace
> every aspect of the entire group of mountains is not because it refers only
> to one small section of the whole (like one square of a chessboard in rela-
> tion to the rest), but because it only relates to a single perspective. The
> sum total of all these various aspects can only be grasped through an act of
> intelligence which links together all the possible perceptions by means of
> operations. . . . Thus the perspective system which the child builds up is
> not perceptual but conceptual in character.[8]

Once this skill reaches full development, the coordination of
perspectives works so automatically in a person's mind that there is
little appreciation for what is taking place. This is another example
of the way spatial ability appears to develop and operate so intuitive-
ly that there is little necessity for most people to take note of its complexity.

Euclidean Space

In spite of the way different points of view affect how objects appear to us, the characteristics of the objects themselves tend to be
preserved. A square looks like an elongated rectangle when it is seen

sideways from one corner. But no matter how the appearance of an object might be effected by the perspective we see it from, objects retain properties that we come to understand as being inherent to them. The square, for example, has four right angles and four equal sides, and it has opposite sides that are parallel to each other. This is true even when we are looking at the square sideways from a corner, and it doesn't appear to be so. Euclidean understanding of space involves knowing when a few rather special properties occur and when these properties are preserved in the structure of objects. These are the properties with which we are all familiar from the study of geometry: parallelism, size of angles, perpendicularity, distances, and arcs. Before these properties are dealt with in geometry, children have usually developed a practical sense of them. This practical knowledge guides children in dealing with geometrically shaped objects, even when the nature of the knowledge cannot be talked about with any precision.

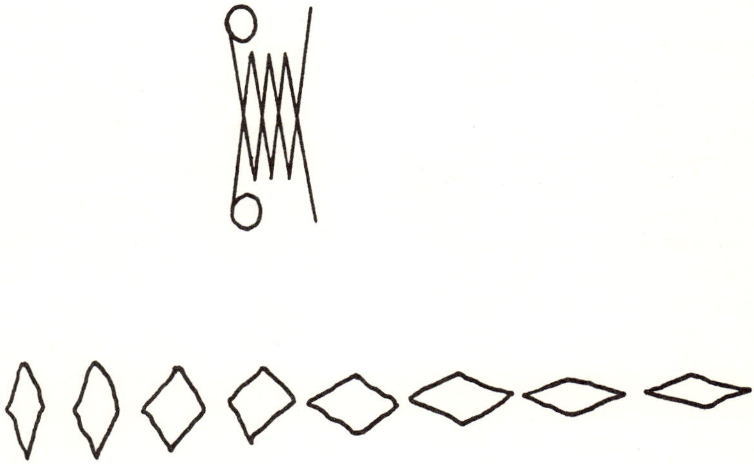

Figure 2-4. At the top is a diagram of "lazy tongs" with the handles as far apart as possible. At the bottom is the somewhat perfected attempt of a child to draw a progression of diamond- or rhombus-shaped holes that the child imagines might be seen as the tongs are pressed together. From J. Piaget and B. Inhelder, *The Child's Conception of Space,* 1967. Reprinted by permission of Humanities Press Inc., Atlantic Highlands, N.J. 07716 and Routledge & Kegan Paul Ltd., London, England.

In one experiment, Piaget showed children a pair of "lazy tongs" in a position with the handles as far apart as possible as shown in the top of Figure 2-4. They were asked to notice the diamond- or rhombus-shaped holes in the tongs and then to show what the holes would look like if the handles were pressed together like a pair of scissors. After some demonstration of changing the extent to which the tongs were open or closed, the children were asked to draw a series of illustrations that would represent the shape of the holes going from the original position to the opposite position in which the handles of the tongs were completely together. In other words, an ideal response might look like that in the bottom of Figure 2-4.

Certain geometric relationships are preserved in the holes as the positioning is changed. Opposite sides are parallel to each other. The lengths of all the sides remain the same and equal to each other. Opposite angles are equal. To the extent that children recognize the need to preserve these relationships while at the same time changing positions of the shapes of the diamonds, they will be able to carry out the exercise with accuracy. Let's look at how this knowledge develops.

Under age four, children are generally unable to draw anything resembling a diamond. Around age five, they can draw a credible diamond when following a model that is in front of them. When the child is asked to anticipate beyond what he can see, it becomes obvious that he has no knowledge of the relationships inherent in the nature of the tongs. The child's anticipations are generally toward bigger holes as the positioning of the tongs changes. The child might say that "they'll get bigger, bigger, bigger,"[9] and the resulting drawings might look like the top sequence in Figure 2-5. "The child cannot anticipate the changes that will occur until he has actually seen them. . . . Once the initial transformation is perceived, it is simply repeated in imagination, whence the idea of the indefinite enlargement of the 'windows,' regardless of the fixed length of their sides."[10]

Around age six, the child begins to anticipate in rather gross ways the direction of the shape of the holes as the tongs are changed. The child may see that the internal area of the diamonds will get larger up to a midpoint in the process and then smaller. But the child tends not to preserve the parallelness of opposite sides or the equality of the lengths of sides. The child's drawing might look like the bottom sequence in Figure 2-5. The child still doesn't grasp the real transformations that are taking place, i.e. the changes of angles within a rigid structure that preserves lengths of sides and parallelism.

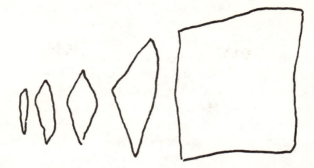

Figure 2-5. Early attempts to draw the progression of diamond- or rhombus-shaped holes in the lazy tongs before the child has acquired such concepts as constancy of length, equality of angles, and parallelism. From J. Piaget and B. Inhelder, *The Child's Conception of Space,* 1967. Reprinted by permission of Humanities Press Inc., Atlantic Highlands, N.J. 07716 and Routledge & Kegan Paul Ltd., London, England.

> The child can imagine the increase and decrease in the surfaces, but only in an overall global fashion. They appear to him, not as a continuous series of transformations, but as abrupt, disjointed changes. . . . In short, the child's reactions show that at this level he anticipates the course of the transformations through a more or less continuous chain of ideas, though not yet by means of operational thought. It is precisely this lack of operations which is responsible for the disjointed character of the changes which he anticipates, and for the fact that the sides of his rhombuses are still neither parallel nor of a constant length.[11]

At about age seven or eight, children begin to construct a fairly accurate series of diamonds that show a preservation in the length of sides and a preservation of parallelism. The children describe their thoughts in various ways: "The rods are always the same. . . . The height gets smaller but the length gets bigger. . . . That one is all right because both sides are sloping the same. . . . It won't get any bigger, only narrower. . . . You can't go any further, it gets completely flat."

Once this operational thinking has been established, the child is ready to work with relationships in geometric figures. The child comes to formal geometric studies with an already established ability to deal with Euclidean relationships, even though the child often times cannot verbally explain his operational understanding.

For research purposes, Piaget pursued a separate understanding of topological space, projective space, and Euclidean space. It is obvious, of course, that there is actually only one space and that these are three interrelated ways by which human intelligence attempts to grasp the patterns and connections in that one space. As our eyes dart around the world about us, visual perception by itself gives us little basis for understanding how that world works. Mature understanding evolves when operationally guided manipulation of the objects of the world and coordination of that manipulation with vision have resulted in knowledge of topological relationships, have provided a child with the capacity to imagine any of the infinite possible perspectives, and have resulted in the recognition of Euclidean relationships. When all three of these can be related to each other to achieve a connected understanding, then a child is prepared to exercise well developed spatial ability.

At the beginning of this chapter, it was suggested that spatial understanding is based on grasping the consistency in relationships between objects as these relationships occur in the context of fluid, changing patterns. If we look at a block with patterns on it and then are asked to draw a picture of the block in some other position conjured up from our imaginations, it is topological understanding, projective understanding, and Euclidean understanding that, working together, allow us to do a credible job.

PSYCHOMETRIC UNDERSTANDING OF SPATIAL ABILITIES

Developmental psychologists like Piaget have made valuable contributions to our understanding of the nature of spatial ability by focusing on the basic skills involved and by describing the way these skills develop in children. Other psychologists, those who use and create tests, look at spatial ability somewhat differently. They are interested in looking at the variation in performance of a wide range of children on the same tasks. In their tests, they usually employ tasks that require a somewhat developed spatial ability and that tap understanding of topological relationships, projective relationships, and Euclidean relationships all at the same time.

In spite of the wide variety of spatial test activities that are in use, psychologists generally agree that they fall into two or three different types. Although Mark McGee, in his recent review, groups spatial tasks into two types,[12] J.W. French, in his earlier study, arrived at a more satisfactory grouping based on three categories.[13] I will follow the French approach and group spatial tests into three categories: (1) pattern arrangement, (2) transformation of orientation, and (3) pattern transformation.

Pattern Arrangement

French's Definition
> An ability to perceive spatial patterns accurately and to compare them with each other.

Guilford's Definition
> An ability to determine relationships between different spatially arranged stimuli and responses and the comprehension of the arrangement of elements within a visual stimulus pattern.[14]

This involves recognizing the relationships between all of the parts of a whole static pattern, so that the pattern can be perceived as a whole and discriminated from other patterns. A rather simple test activity might require a person to complete a graphic pattern where the completion is clearly implied by the consistencies in the parts of the pattern that are given (Figure 2-6). In this type of activity, it is assumed that the patterns are being seen from approximately the same perspective and that no transformation of orientation has taken place in any of the patterns.

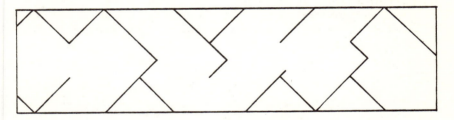

Figure 2-6. Find the consistencies in the pattern so that it can be completed.

Transformation of Orientation

French's Definition
> An ability to remain unconfused by the varying orientation in which a spatial pattern may be presented.

Thurstone's Definition
> An ability to recognize the identity of an object when it is seen

from different angles or an ability to visualize a rigid configuration when it is moved into different positions. An ability to think about those spatial relations in which the body orientation of the observer is an essential part of the problem. [15]

This type of activity assumes the prior ability of recognizing pattern arrangement. It requires that a person see that the same pattern arrangements are being maintained, even if they are seen from a different direction or angle. In transformation of orientation activities, the parts of the pattern or object itself remain rigid. It is the angle of perspective of the observer that changes. Shepard and Metzler have created tasks that require people to determine if two cubic structures are identical except for being rotated to be seen from a different direction (Figure 2-7). [16] This kind of activity requires either the imagined rotation of an object in one's mind or it requires imagining oneself placed in a different position in relation to the object.

Pattern Transformation

Thurstone's Definition
> An ability to visualize a configuration in which there is movement or displacement among the internal parts of the configuration.

Guilford's Definition
> An ability to imagine . . . the folding or unfolding of flat patterns. . . . The motion of machinery. . . . Tests that present a stimulus pictorially and in which some manipulation or transformation to another visual arrangement is involved. [17]

This kind of task assumes the skills already involved in pattern arrangement and transformation of orientation. It adds the requirement of understanding how the parts of objects can change position in relation to each other and yet not violate the way the pattern hangs together. The classic example is the visualized paper folding task in which a person must anticipate what a pattern will look like when it is folded. In Figure 2-8, could the house on the left be constructed from folding the pattern on the right? If you carry out the mental manipulation of this pattern, you can see that the color arrangement of the house is not consistent with that of the pattern. This kind of task is quite difficult for many people. When

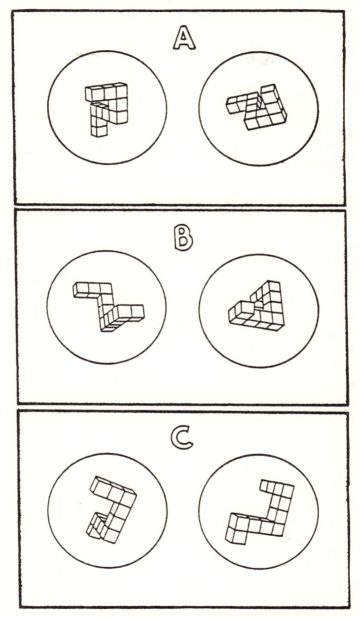

Figure 2-7. The pairs of block structures in A and B are the same except for being rotated to a different position in three-dimentional space. The pair of structures in C are not the same. From R. Shepard and J. Metzler, Mental rotation of three-dimensional objects, *Science, 171:*701-703, February 1971. Copyright 1971 by the American Association for the Advancement of Science. Courtesy of R. Shepard and J. Metzler and *Science.*

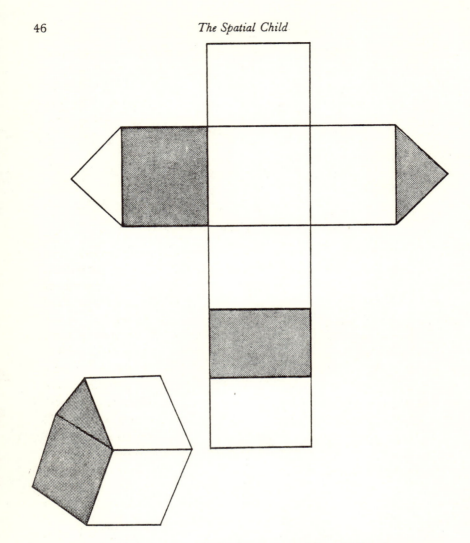

Figure 2-8. Could the house on the left be constructed from folding the paper pattern on the right?

psychometricians present this kind of activity to even mature adults, definite distinctions between people who have considerable spatial ability and those who do not begin to emerge.

DOES SPATIAL TESTING HAVE ANYTHING TO DO WITH THE REAL WORLD?

Review of spatial test items like those above might lead to some skepticism. One might ask if these activities involve anything of real importance. If a child performs well on spatial testing tasks, does it mean anything other than he did well on spatial testing tasks? In research terms one would ask about what the predictive validity of these tests is; i.e. if you know a child has high scores on a spatial test, is there anything else you can predict from this with some degree of accuracy? Most importantly, what can you predict about the school performance of a child, and what can you predict about the child's performance in the "real world" after leaving school? Some interesting research on the predictive validity of spatial testing has been done.

One extensive study was conducted over a number of years in the late 1930s and early 1940s. Frank Holliday, a trainer of engineering apprentices in England, administered a battery of eight spatial and mechanical ability tests to students.[18] He also administered a test of verbal intelligence to the same students. After these students had participated in courses in mechanical drawing, he asked the instructors of the courses to rank the students according to the order of their merit. He could then study the relationship between their performance in the courses and their scores on the tests. Holliday found a rather substantial relationship. Those students who performed well on the tests also performed well in the mechanical drawing classes. In statistical terms, the correlation between the two was $+.67$. ($+1.00$ is a perfect direct relationship, $.00$ is no relationship, and -1.00 is a perfect opposite relationship.)

It would, of course, be possible to say that students who are intelligent and work hard will tend to do well whether they are performing on a battery of tests or performing in a mechanical drawing class. One would expect a positive relationship between any test and school performance. Holliday had covered this possibility by administering a verbal intelligence test. He found that there was virtually no relationship between the verbal test scores and student performance in mechanical drawing. The correlation was $+.07$, indicating that the spatial tests were about 100 times (statistically speaking, $R_s^2 = .45$, $R_v^2 = .005$) more predictive of success in mechanical drawing than was the verbal test. One would conclude that the spatial tests were predictive not simply because they required concentration and intelligence. Their predictive value derived from the fact that the spatial tests were assessing skills that are important in mechanical drawing, while the verbal test was not.

The most impressive part of Frank Holliday's study is that he followed these students after they completed school to see how they performed in the real world of engineering. In one study he waited until a group of ninety-one engineers had been on the job for at least two years.[19] Then he asked the supervisors of these former students to rate their job performance as being either above average, average, or below average. Holliday also divided the former students into three groups according to whether they were high, average, or low in their original performance on the spatial tests. The number of former students falling into each category of the two-way classification is shown in Table 2-I. After looking at this relationship between test performance and engineering performance, one could conclude that students who did well on the spatial tests were not likely to fail on the job. Those who did poorly on the tests were in substantial risk of failing on the job. One could say that this testing could be of considerable value in counseling students concerning their prospects and risks in entering the engineering field. Considering that most of these engineers must have had some inclination toward mechanical skills before entering school, it is rather impressive that Holliday was able to make these distinctions.

Table 2-I

Holliday Results Indicating Numbers of Engineers Grouped
by Scores on Spatial Tests and Also by Engineering Performance

On the Job Engineering Performance	Spatial Test Performance		
	High	Average	Low
Above Average	15	10	3
Average	8	17	11
Below Average	5	9	13

Another way of looking at the predictive validity of spatial tests is to determine whether their predictive value is specific to areas of achievement that seem logically related to spatial ability. On the other hand, are they predictive of all sorts of achievement? If so, then they give little guidance concerning the direction in which spatial abilities can most profitably be applied. There is nothing in the Holliday research that indicates that spatial testing would not be just as predictive of performance in learning a foreign language as performance in engineering.

In the 1940s, Karl Holzinger and Frances Swineford carried on research at the University of Minnesota that answers this question. They administered spatial ability tests to 174 high school students and also collected information on how these students were performing in a variety of subject areas.[20] Holzinger and Swineford found that the spatial tests were highly predictive of success in drawing and also had good predictive value of performance in shop and crafts. The tests were of some value in predicting performance in plane geometry, history, and chemistry. On the other hand, the spatial tests were of no value in predicting performance in biology, English, or foreign language. In fact, there was a slight negative relationship between test scores and performance in foreign language; the better a student did on the tests, the worse he performed in foreign language. The actual correlations between tests scores and school performance in the various areas are as follows:

Drawing	+ .69
Shop and Crafts	+ .46
Chemistry	+ .26
History	+ .24
Plane Geometry	+ .23
Biology	.00
English	.00
Foreign Language	− .06

The pattern in these relationships seems to be that the more a school subject area depends on the memorization and appropriate use of words or verbal terms, the less valuable spatial testing is in predicting success. On the other hand, the more a subject area stresses visualized manipulation of objects in space or stresses the understanding of relationships in broad and general patterns, the more valuable the spatial tests are in predicting success. One could say that this is a rather logical, expected outcome. The correlations with history and with geometry might be considered exceptions to this rule. However, in spite of the verbal nature of history, to the extent that it presents broad patterns of connected information, it tends to be appreciated by children who are dominant in spatial skills. History was a favorite subject of both Einstein and Newton when they were children. Plane geometry is very spatial in nature and therefore might be expected to have a somewhat higher correlation with spatial tests. However, it should be remembered that formal proofs in plane geometry are highly verbal in nature.

The Holliday studies and the Holzinger and Swineford studies provide confidence that it is appropriate to deal with human abilities in a differentiated way. This should help us refrain from the common abuse of expecting some children to do well in all subject areas and others to do poorly in all areas. We are in the position of saying with some certainty that spatial tests do tap something special in the mental processes of children. By being in tune to the exceptional presence of strong spatial skills in some children, we are more likely to guide them toward experiences that will take full advantage of their capabilities.

REFERENCES

1. Piaget, J., and Inhelder, B. *The Child's Conception of Space.* New York: Norton and Co., 1967, p. 30.
2. *Ibid.,* p. 35.
3. *Ibid.,* p. 36.
4. *Ibid.,* pp. 36-37.
5. *Ibid.,* pp. 215-222.
6. *Ibid.,* p. 225.
7. *Ibid.,* p. 240.
8. *Ibid.,* pp. 244-245.
9. *Ibid.,* p. 309.
10. *Ibid.,* pp. 309-310.
11. *Ibid.,* p. 313
12. McGee, M.G. Human spatial abilities: psychometric studies and environmental, genetic, hormonal, and neurological influences. *Psychological Bulletin, 86*:889-919, 1979.
13. French, J.W. The description of aptitude and achievement tests in terms of rotated factors. *Psychometric Monographs* (No. 5). Chicago: University of Chicago Press, 1951.
14. McGee, *op. cit.,* p. 891.
15. McGee, *op. cit.,* p. 891.

16. Shepard, R.N., and Metzler, J. Mental rotation of three-dimensional objects. *Science, 171*:701-703, 1971.

17. McGee, *op. cit.,* p. 891.

18. Holliday, F. A study into the selection of apprentices for the engineering industry. *Occupational Psychology, 14*:69-81, 1940.

19. Holliday, F. The relations between psychological test scores and subsequent job proficiency in the engineering industry. *Occupational Psychology, 17*:168-185, 1943.

20. Holzinger, K.J., and Swineford, F. The relation of two bi-factors to achievement in geometry and other subjects. *The Journal of Educational Psychology, 37*:263, 1946.

Chapter 3

THE RESEARCH CONVERGES

INFORMATION PROCESSING RESEARCH

PERHAPS throughout human history there have been those who took note in an informal way that some of their craftier friends had trouble explaining in words the nifty things they could do. This is a common observation that can be made by anyone who is sensitive to it. The opposite pattern is also commonly observed: Some people have great facility in the use of language but little sense of the relationships between objects in the world around them. These, of course, are not the only two possible patterns. Most people seem to have a good balance between language skills and spatial skills. There are the truly blest who possess both in large quantity. It is the minority of people who have a distinctly unbalanced relationship between the two.

The formal study of relationships between skill patterns started in England in the late 1800s, and, as is usual in most areas of study, it started with vague intuitions and outright confusion. Sir Francis Galton, one of the forefathers of the study of differences in human abilities, seemed to have spatial giftedness much in mind when he wrote his *Inquiries into Human Faculty and Its Development*. Galton was undoubtedly convinced that the possession of clear imagery of the external world and of the ability to create images in one's mind even when the imagined objects are not present is crucial for scientific work. Sir Francis Galton* made up a short questionnaire and sent it around to some of his friends in the world of science. His questionnaire said —

> Before addressing yourself to any of the questions on the opposite page, think of some definite object — suppose it is your breakfast-table as you sat down to it this morning — and consider carefully the picture that rises before your mind's eye. . . .
>
> 1. Illumination — Is the image dim or fairly clear? Is its brightness com-

---

*From Frances Galton, *Inquiries into Human Faculty and its Development*, 1973. Courtesy of J. M. Dent & Sons Ltd., London, England.

parable to that of the actual scene?

2. Definition — Are all of the objects pretty well defined at the same time, or is the place of sharpest definition at any one moment more contracted than it is a real scene?

3. Colouring — Are the colours of the china, of the toast, bread-crust, mustard, meat, parsley, or whatever may have been on the table, quite distinct and natural?[1]

Although Sir Francis found that some of his scientific friends had the capacity for vivid imagery, most did not, and some seemed to be almost totally devoid of such thought processes. He said, "To my astonishment, I found that the great majority of the men of science to whom I first applied protested that mental imagery was unknown to them. . . . They had no more notion of its nature than a colour-blind man, who had not discerned his defect, has of the nature of colour. They had a mental deficiency of which they were unaware, and naturally enough supposed that those who affirmed they possessed it, were romancing."[2]

Galton experienced further astonishment when he interviewed a number of people who were not in any way distinguished for their scientific thinking. Many of them claimed to experience much more vivid mental imagery than did the scientists. He knew something was wrong with his original hypothesis. Being one of England's most brilliant men of the late 1800s, he immediately found a way to reorganize his thinking so that it would fit the newly discovered facts. Now instead of suggesting that vivid imagery was important to scientific thought, he suggested that scientific work had negative effects upon imagery. He concludes "that an over-ready perception of sharp mental pictures is antagonistic to the acquirement of habits of highly-generalized and abstract thought, especially when the steps of reasoning are carried on by words as symbols, and that if the faculty of seeing the pictures was ever possessed by men who think hard, it is very apt to be lost by disuse."[3]

In his confusion, Galton seemed to have jumped from one extreme position to the opposite; from expecting scientific thinkers to have vivid imagery to expecting them to have little imagery. In the process of doing so, he had one passing intuition that seems to anticipate current thought on spatial ability. He was still sure that scientists need some special way of thinking about the objects in the world, and he attempted to say what that was.

I am, however, bound to say, that the missing faculty (vivid imagery) seems to be replaced so serviceably by other modes of conception, chiefly, I believe, connected with the incipient motor sense, not of the eyeballs only but of the muscles generally, that men who declare themselves entirely deficient in the power of seeing mental pictures can nevertheless give life-like descriptions of what they have seen, and can otherwise express themselves as if they were gifted with a vivid visual imagination.[4]

Galton may have come to realize that the basis for spatial understanding is not so much the picture-like imagining of the environment, as it is the systematic manipulation of that environment. As understood in Piaget's line of research, manipulation of the environment eventually leads to concrete operations and then to formal, abstract operations. Formal operations are the basis for relational understanding of the spatial world. Thus, the abstracted relational thought that derives from manipulation of objects of the world is more fundamental to spatial ability than is picture-like imagery. For example an understanding of how the infinitely possible lines of sight relate to each other is an abstraction from the world as we see it, and realization of this abstraction cannot be achieved without acting in relation to the environment.

This review of Galton's progression in thinking is of instructional value. Many researchers have made the mistake of equating vivid pictorial imagery with spatial thinking. Spatial thinking certainly involves a certain kind of imagery. But it isn't so much an exact pictorial imagery as it is an imagery that takes relational aspects of the physical world and focuses on these aspects rather independently of the remaining details. In this way, the selected relational aspects can come to be thoroughly understood. The way Albert Einstein described his own thought processes is perhaps an approximation of what is involved.

> The psychological entities which seem to serve as elements in thought are certain signs and more or less clear images which can be voluntarily reproduced and combined. . . . It is also clear that the desire to arrive finally at logically connected concepts is the emotional basis of this rather vague play with the above mentioned elements. . . . This combinatory play seems to be the essential feature in productive thought. . . . The above mentioned elements are in my case visual and some of muscular type.[5]

The most profound spatial thought processes do not so much involve picture-like imagery as they involve abstracted, relational, manipulative imagery.

Many years after Galton pursued his speculations, Anne Roe, in the 1940s, conducted studies that helped clear up some of the confusion.[6] She interviewed a large number of scientists. Rather than asking Galton's "breakfast-table" question, Anne Roe used a different approach in which she was probing for various kinds of imagery. First, she asked the scientists to describe the form in which their thoughts occurred. Then she asked more specifically about their use of visual imagery. Here again, she left things wide open by suggesting different possibilities — concrete, diagrammatic, symbolic, three dimensional and freely manipulable. Anne Roe not only found considerable use of visual imagery among the scientists, she also found some interesting patterns. There was a variety of imagery used by the various scientists, but there was a distinct tendency for the physical scientists and the social scientists to go in two distinct directions. The physical scientists tended to use visual imagery and visual symbolization, while the social scientists used verbal imagery and verbal symbolization. The numbers of each kind of scientist who could be described in these ways are given in Table 3-I.

Table 3-I

Roe's Findings on the Tendencies of Physical Scientists
and Social Scientists to Use Either Visual or Verbal Imagery

Type of Scientist	Type of Imagery and Symbolization	
	Visual	Verbal
Biologists and physicists	20	8
Psychologists and anthropologists	2	11

Anne Roe also offers some interesting observations on the deviant cases, i.e. physical scientists who tended toward the verbal mode and social scientists who tended toward the visual mode. "Subjects who do not follow the pattern most typical for their own group are also somewhat less like their colleagues in their work and personalities."[7] Among the physical scientists, those who tended toward the verbal mode had, during their school days, shown considerable interest in the classics and literature, as is typical of social scientists. The two social scientists who tended toward the visual mode had never shown interest in the classics or literature at any age. In this research, Anne Roe helped to correct Sir Francis Galton's mistake. She demonstrated that a more abstracted form of visual imagery does seem to play its role in professions that rely on an understanding of spatial relationships. One simply needs to move beyond the expectation of picture-like imagery.

In the effort to make clear the distinction between simple pictorial imagery and spatial thinking, perhaps another distinction would be helpful. Some thought processes seem to involve the faithful reproduction of detailed information. Other thought processes involve abstracted transformations of information based on understanding of relationships. Visualization is important in spatial thinking, but to the extent that it only involves the faithful recognition of detailed information, visualization does not involve spatial ability. Spatial ability also involves understanding of relationships in patterns such that manipulative, operational thought can take place. This is necessary for analyzing structural relationships, for recognizing analogous situations in information, and for creating appropriate new syntheses of information. Spatial thought goes far beyond simple pictorial imagery. Ways of thinking might first be distinguished as either verbal or visual. Secondly, these thought processes can be distinguished as emphasizing either direct memory or relational thought. Spatial thinking occurs when visualization and relational thought are applied together. When the same distinction is made in verbal thinking, the diagram in Table 3-II is the result.

Whereas Roe and Galton focused on the mental processes of accomplished scientists, during the 1930s another line of research that made similar distinctions in more average populations began. In one study, an English psychologist by the name of Bartlett had people carry out tasks and describe the mental strategies they used. He had people associate figural patterns with words.[8] For example the symbols $>X<$ might be associated with the word *conversation*. People were given a list of these figure-word associations and then asked to remember them. When they were asked to describe the strategies by which this task was carried out, two patterns emerged. There were visual thinkers who tended to make associations through visual patterns. For example the openness of the letter *c* in *conversation* might be

Table 3-II

Types of Thought Processes
Classified by Level and Mode

Level of Thought Process	Mode of Thought Process	
	Visual	Verbal
Memory	Picture-like imagery	Exact verbal memory
Relational Thought	Manipulation of spatial relationships	Manipulation of symbolic relationships

associated with the openness of the $>$ and $<$ signs and thus might become the key for reproducing the association. There were also verbal thinkers. The verbal thinker might call the pattern the "greater than, less than complex" and use that name to remember the association. Although many of Bartlett's subjects could on occasion use either a visual or verbal strategy, he found that most subjects tended to use one dominant strategy on most occasions. They could thus justifiably be called visualizers and verbalizers. And since the visualizers were going beyond a pictorial recognition of information and relying on sensitivity to patterns in the information, we could say the visualizers were using spatial strategies.

Following in this information-processing tradition, in 1960, Clementina Kuhlman reported on a dissertation study she conducted at Harvard University. The purpose of the study was to determine how a visual learning style relates to the way children learn in school. Fortunately, for current interests, Kuhlman used a spatial relations test as the means of determining who the visual children were. Observations were made on two groups of children. The first visual-spatial group achieved high scores on spatial tests but lower scores on language tests. The second verbal group achieved high scores on language tests but low scores on spatial tests.[9] Kuhlman found that the two groups of children tended to do superior work on different sorts of tasks. Verbal children tended to do well on tasks that require a sensitivity to the conventional, culturally understood, functional qualities of things. For example a ball, a balloon, and a hula hoop would be linked together on the basis that they are all toys. Visual-spatial children, on the other hand, tend to associate things on the basis of recognizing patterns in their physical qualities. The ball, balloon, and hula hoop would be associated on the basis of being round. One could say that verbal children are culturally sensitive, while spatial children are physically sensitive. Verbal children do well when conventional understanding is important, while spatial children do well when being aware of physical properties and patterns in things is important.

Research that establishes the distinction between those who rely most heavily on verbal cognitive strategies and those who rely most heavily on visual-spatial cognitive strategies has continued to the present time.[10] Perhaps the most significant, current information-processing research has been conducted by MacLeod at the University of Washington and by Sternberg at Yale University.[11] In the research at the University of Washington, somewhat traditional, but simplified, reading comprehension tasks are used. First, a subject is asked to read a sentence such as "Plus is above star," and then is shown a picture that represents that the statement is true or a picture that indicates the statement is false (i.e. a star above a plus or a plus above a star). The subject is then asked to indicate whether the statement is true or false. In this type of research the primary interest focuses on two lengths of time. The first is the length of time it takes a person to comprehend the sentence. This is called comprehension time. The second is the length of time it takes a person to look at the picture and to confirm that the statement is true or false. This is called verification time. This kind of activity can be done on a computer terminal so that the subjects can push a button when they are ready to read a new sentence, push a second button when they are ready to look at the picture, and then push a third button to confirm truth or falsehood. In this way, the exact comprehension time and verification time can easily be measured.

The most interesting result of this research is that two distinct patterns seemed to emerge. The larger group of subjects took approximately the same amount of time to read the sentences and to verify the pictures. A second, and smaller, group of subjects took a much longer amount of time to comprehend the sentences, but a much shorter amount of time to verify the pictures. The average amount of time for each group on each part is given in Table 3-III. Colin MacLeod and his colleagues concluded that whereas the first

Table 3-III

MacLeod's Results Showing Average Amount of Time It
Takes Two Groups to Comprehend a Sentence and Then to
Verify that It Does or Does Not Describe a Picture

Groups	Length of Time in Seconds	
	Comprehension	Verification
Verbal coders	1.65	1.21
Spatial coders	2.60	.65

group was carrying the reading information from the first part of the task to the second in a verbal code, the second group was translating the reading information into a spatial image before they moved on to the second part of the task. The spatial image took longer to create because it was in a different mode than the reading material, but once this mode was achieved, it was much easier for these subjects to match the spatial images with the pictures. Reading comprehension thus took much longer, but verification a much shorter time. Robert Sternberg has achieved similar results with other kinds of tasks.

The MacLeod and Sternberg findings raise some interesting questions concerning those who could be called spatial coders. Are these people particularly debilitated under speed-reading conditions because they need to immediately transform verbal information to a spatial code? If they are particularly debilitated, are there ways they can be helped to adapt? Are there ways in which school teachers should change instructional strategies to help children who rely primarily on spatial coding of information?

DIVIDING TEST SCORES

While some psychologists like Bartlett, Kuhlman, and MacLeod have concentrated on studying information processing on distinct activities, other psychologists have been interested in looking at the way scores derived from a variety of ability tests hang together in groups. This second group of psychologists is interested in finding out what happens when a number of different kinds of tests are administered to the same children. They wonder if all of the tests go together; i.e. if a child achieves a high score on one test, will he tend to get high scores on all other tests without much difference between tests? Or will there be certain groups of tests that go together and that do not have scores that correspond with other groups of tests? In order to study this question with some mathematical precision, psychologists developed a rather complex statistical technique called factor analysis, so complex that certain aspects of factor analysis are clouded in controversy to this day. As it happens, one of the controversies involves the distinction between verbal ability and spatial ability.

One of the assumptions involved in using factor analysis to study test scores is that there are certain underlying aspects of human ability that determine how well a given person performs on different tests. These aspects of ability result in the factors derived from factor analysis. It is assumed that different children possess different amounts of each ability. Likewise, it is assumed that different tests require different amounts of each ability for maximum performance. The score that a child receives on a given test is then considered to be determined by the extent to which the child possesses the underlying abilities required for performing well on the given test.

Working from these assumptions, if one gives a number of different tests that require varying amounts of different underlying abilities to a number of children who possess varying amounts of these underlying abilities, one should be able to get a hint of the patterns in the underlying abilities. This is done by deriving what are called factor loadings. Factor loadings are somewhat like correlation coefficients in that they indicate the extent to which a given test is dependent on a given ability factor. Like correlation coefficients, they tend to range between + 1.00 and − 1.00. If two tests have opposite signs for their loadings on the same factor, this could be interpreted as meaning that the factor in some sense is causing the scores on these tests to go in opposite directions. For example, if Test I has a loading of + .63 and Test II has a loading of − .47 on the same factor, it could be said that whereas some people will tend to have higher scores on one test, other people will tend to have higher scores on the other test, and the two groups of people will tend to be somewhat distinct.

This, of course, is an oversimplification. When many tests are administered to the same children and two or more factors are derived from these test scores, the patterns that cause some scores to be high and others low are intertwined in such a way that one cannot actually observe the uncontaminated effects of one factor on the scores. Also, all ability test scores tend to vary together such that all scores for a given person tend to be in the same magnitude. This tendency for the scores of a given individual to be in approximately the same magnitude is given a special name *g*, which means general intellectual ability.

When factor analysis is carried out, factors are found one at a time and in order. The first factor derived is representative of *g*, or the tendency of all test scores for a given child to be relatively high or low together. When the first factor or *g* is found, the factor loadings indicate the extent to which each test goes along with or is loaded on *g*. The scores on some tests will be largely determined by *g*, and others will be less determined by *g*. However, because *g* is the tendency for all test scores to be somewhat of the same magnitude, the signs for the loadings on *g* will all be positive. The resulting factor loadings for the first factor in a study conducted by El Koussy are given in Table 3-IV.[12]

Table 3-IV

First Factor Loadings from
a Study by El Koussy

Tests	First Factor Loadings on *g*
Pattern perception	+ .76
Correlate education B	+ .65
Form relations	+ .43
Spatial analogies	+ .63
Drawing	+ .40

After deriving the first or *g* factor, a psychologist is prepared to go on to look at the second factor. With traditional factor-analytic procedures, factor loadings on the second and subsequent factors are bound to go both in the positive and negative directions. Because the derivation of the *g* factor has taken account of the tendency for all test scores for an individual to be somewhat of the same magnitude, subsequent factors will naturally be looking at the remaining tendencies of different tests to not be of the same magnitude for separate groups of children. If we didn't find these additional tendencies, factor analysis would be of no value. We would only be able to conclude that people are either intelligent in every way or dull in every way and that there is nothing else to be discovered. The world is more interesting than that.

In many early factor-analytic studies, when the second factor was derived, it appeared that tests of a spatial nature would tend to group together in one direction, while verbal tests would group together in the opposite direction. This can be seen in the results from a dissertation study done by Clarke at London University (Table 3-V).[13]

Table 3-V

Second Factor Loadings
from a Study by Clarke

Tests	Second *k/v* Factor Loadings
Spatial Tests	
Noughts and crosses	+ .44
Designs	+ .38
Line pattern	+ .38
Clock face	+ .35
Form relations	+ .27
Dot series	+ .21
Reversals and inversions	+ .21
Incomplete drawings	+ .20
Fitting shapes	+ .20
Ball	+ .20
Nonverbal selection	+ .17
Verbal Tests	
Verbal analogies I	− .14
Selection	− .15
Verbal analogies II	− .23
Verbal fours	− .25
Best answers	− .31
Inferences	− .33
Disarranged sentences	− .52

It is very clear in this second factor result that the spatial tests are grouped together and tend to go in one direction, while the verbal tests are grouped together and go in the opposite direction. There were many early factor-analytic studies that arrived at somewhat similar results.[14] This kind of result came to be known as a bipolar factor because it implied that certain skills tend to be in opposition to each other. At various points there were attempts to make psychological sense of this bipolar factor. It was sometimes called the *k/v* factor; *k* representing *kinesthetic imagery* or *spatial ability,* and *v* representing *verbal ability*. The *k/v* implies that both were being measured on the same factor, but at opposite ends of the bipolar factor.

This result would indicate that, to the extent the second factor determines the magnitude of test scores, if a person had strength in one type of ability, this would in some way be associated with a weakness in the other. Everyone knew, of course, that this was not entirely the way things worked. The first *g* factor was the most dominant factor in all studies. The level of performance on all tests had, therefore, to correspond to some degree. It seemed feasible, however, that there might be certain elements of performance on spatial tests and elements of performance on verbal tests that might be naturally antagonistic to each other. In her 1936 London University dissertation, Clarke suggested that verbal skills and spatial imagery skills were inversely related to one another.[13] There were times during the 1930s and 1940s when this kind of result was taken to have implications for the way children should be selected for different kinds of schooling. This was especially true in Britain.

But as the bipolar interpretation began to be seriously considered, it also became a source of controversy. Lewis Thurstone, the most eminent of American factor analysts during the 1930s, had doubts about the appropriateness of trying to interpret bipolar solutions. In 1934, he declared that intellectual abilities exist in nature in a "positive manifold."[16] What he seemed to mean by this is that the ability traits of people that result in factor scores may be present in varying amounts, but only in a positive direction. The idea of below zero intelligence in one of these underlying traits is not reasonable. Therefore, when we attempt to interpret bipolar factors, we are really looking at two or more aspects of intelligence that are being measured on the same factor. Thurstone insisted that if we want to

identify distinct separate traits, factor-analytic methods must be adjusted so that the traits tend to be manifested in separate factors and
always in a positive direction.

This seemed to be a reasonable assertion. It is interesting,
however, when rigorous, mathematically minded scientists like
Thurstone make rather philosophical assertions about the nature of
things, assertions aren't always based on information collected, but
rather on the way they think things should be. Thurstone's assertion
of the "positive manifold" might have been reasonable, but it might
also have caused Thurstone and many other psychologists to
overlook the meaningfulness of information sitting right in front of
them. Research in the areas of information processing, cerebral
asymmetry, and learning disabilities would later establish the importance of looking for oppositional elements in verbal and spatial
ability, but factor-analytic research might well have led the way if it
had not been set off course by Thurstone. Thurstone made revisions
in the methods for carrying out factor analysis. Bipolar factors were
mathematicized out of existence; they violated nature. Because of
Thurstone's eminence as a statistician, his philosophical declaration
was widely accepted, and in the words of Broverman and Klaiber,
"negative relationships among cognitive abilities have not been
seriously considered since."[17]

There has been an undercurrent of dissatisfaction with the
Thurstone solution ever since it was developed. Much of the opposition has come from British psychologists, such as Philip Vernon and
I. MacFarlane Smith. These British psychologists have been interested in the possibility that there are certain aspects of spatial
ability and verbal ability that do run counter to each other. In a
review of biographical literature on men of genius, Smith has taken
note of the tendency for spatial ability and verbal ability to be out of
proportion to the extent that it is appropriate to assert that many
highly accomplished people are specialized in one or the other.[18]
Smith asserts that if this is an important aspect of the way intellectual abilities are actually represented in people, then the second
bipolar factor is meaningful and interpretable and should not be ignored simply because of Thurstone's philosophical assumption.

In his extensive research and writing on spatial ability, Smith's
greatest concern was that the accumulated knowledge was rarely being applied by educators. Yates and Barr had demonstrated that

spatial test scores were much better predictors than any other test scores on how well grammar school students would do in certain technical subject areas.[19] Nisbet and Buchan had found that college-preparatory school entrance exams that were verbally oriented were not predictive at all of how well students would do in later science courses at Aberdeen University; some were negative predictors.[20] In spite of strong evidence for the distinct value of spatial testing, in a survey of British preparatory schools, Smith found that very few schools were using any kind of spatial testing in the selection of students. Because of the lack of such testing, children with exceptional spatial skills tended to be grossly underrepresented in these college-preparatory schools. In Smith's own study, a battery of tests were specially administered to all of the students in two of these schools. It was found that 16 percent of the students had verbal IQs of 134 or above, while only 1 percent had spatial IQ scores that high. It was clear that a rather small portion of the spatially gifted children in Britain were being selected to attend college-preparatory schools. This was true in spite of the evidence that spatial abilities are the best predictors of success in certain areas of study.

Smith was concerned about this problem because a large portion of spatially gifted children were not being admitted to college-preparatory schools, and this made it almost certain that only a small portion of the pool of spatially gifted persons available in this country would reach those technical professions where their ability was most needed and where they would be best adapted psychologically. The pool of spatially gifted children included those children with the greatest potential for significant contributions to engineering, mathematics, and other scientific fields, and the supply of high-quality scientific workers was likely limited by this mistake in admission procedures.[21]

Smith's work on factor analysis and his interest in the bipolar *k/v* factor led to his concern for the way children were being selected for school programs. The information-processing research and the cerebral asymmetry research that has been accumulating since the publication of Smith's extensive study of spatial abilities gives even more weight to the argument that the *k/v* factor provides a meaningful interpretation of differences in human abilities. Perhaps in some limited sense, spatial abilities and verbal abilities are counterproductive to each other; i.e. if a person is particularly strong in one type of ability, this may interfere with his performance in the other area.

In 1969, Donald Broverman and Edward Klaiber, two American psychologists, reported a study in which they were attempting to establish a physiological foundation for the *k/v* interpretation. They, like the British psychologists, were dissatisfied with the Thurstone dictum on the positive manifold and with Thurstone's assertion of the inappropriateness of interpreting the *k/v* factor. They were interested in the effects of the sex hormones estrogen and androgen on an enzyme called monoamine oxidase (MAO). MAO regulates the action of certain neurotransmitters in our brains. Since the sex hormones reduce the effectiveness of MAO, Broverman and Klaiber hypothesized that there should be a difference in cognitive functioning between people who have higher levels of sex hormones and those who have lower levels. More specifically, they differentiated between what they called simple, perceptual-motor skills and more complex, perceptual-restructuring tasks. Those possessing higher levels of the sex hormones were expected to be more specialized for perceptual-motor skills while those possessing lower levels were expected to be more specialized for perceptual-restructuring tasks. The distinction is identical to the verbal-spatial difference in that Broverman and Klaiber used verbal and symbolic coding tests to measure perceptual-motor skills and spatial manipulation tests to measure perceptual-restructuring skills. The hypothesis seemed to be confirmed by their data.[22] Broverman and Klaiber were investigating one possible physiological reason for the *k/v* solution derived from factor analysis. The research that they initiated is being pursued by others, and there are likely to be more definitive answers to their hypothesis in the future.[23] Their research does add another dimension to the effort to understand the relationship between verbal and spatial skills.

THE STRENGTHS OF LEARNING-DISABLED CHILDREN

Any general assertion about learning-disabled children as a group would be inappropriate. Many different learning difficulties come under the umbrella of the learning-disabilities designation, and nothing specific can be said of the group as a whole. There is, however, one group of learning-disabled children who are of special interest to educators of the gifted. These are children who are distinctly deficient in their attempts to learn the basic language skills, but nevertheless above average on indicators of their more general intellectual capabilities.

In a 1965 publication, McLeod, an Australian psychologist, pulled together the results from eight different studies in which disabled readers had been administered the Wechsler Intelligence Scales for Children (WISC). The WISC consists of a collection of twelve subtests and therefore is of special interest to those who are interested in distinguishing between areas of intellectual strength and areas of intellectual weakness in children. In the eight studies reviewed by McLeod, a number of research approaches were used. Sometimes the disabled readers were compared to successful readers and sometimes they were looked at by themselves. When there was a comparison group, sometimes the two groups were matched for overall intelligence and sometimes they were not. Nevertheless, some consistent results were derived.[24]

In each study it was determined whether each given subtest was a strength or a weakness for the disabled readers. For each given subtest there was near total consistency as to whether it came out a strength or a weakness. The summarized results from the eight studies are given in Table 3-VI.

Table 3-VI

McLeod's Review of Studies in which WISC
Subtests Are Found to Be a Strength or
a Weakness for Disabled Readers

WISC Subtests	Number in which Subtest Is a Strength	Number in which Subtest Is a Weakness
Block design	5	0
Picture arrangement	4	0
Comprehension	4	0
Picture completion	3	0
Similarities	3	0
Object assembly	2	0
Vocabulary	2	3
Digit span	0	3
Information	0	6
Arithmetic	0	7
Coding	0	7

Only one subtest shows an inconsistency; this is vocabulary. Vocabulary is a strength for disabled readers in two studies and a weakness in three. The fact that vocabulary would sometimes come out as a strength for disabled readers may seem to be inconsistent with the fact that it is a verbal test. However, the vocabulary subtest is administered by giving words orally and asking a child to give an oral definition. Since giving unmemorized definitions involves cognitive transformations that go far beyond the words involved, perhaps it is not so unusual that it should sometimes be a strength for disabled readers.

The other results are surprisingly consistent. Disabled readers have difficulties with the retention and quick processing of detailed information. For example the coding subtest on which they were most consistently disabled requires that a child quickly memorize a relationship between two different symbol sets (for example, 1 = *, 2 = &, 3 = $, 4 = #), and then quickly transform a series from one set into the other (transform 3, 2, 4, 3, 1, 4). Intellectually, this is the most simplistic of activities. On the other hand, the subtests on which the disabled readers did well all involved the grasp of a gestalt of interconnected, patterned information. The disabled readers were strongest on the block design subtest. This subtest requires a child to use a set of patterned blocks to reproduce a two-dimensional visual pattern. The other thing to notice in McLeod's results is that the spatial tests were consistently a strength for the disabled readers. This would include block design and object assembly, and perhaps it would also include picture completion and picture arrangement.

The disabled readers also did well on the two nonspatial tests; these are comprehension and similarities. Both of these subtests involve high level understanding of relationships and anticipating the implications from these relationships. One might distinguish the tests on which the reading-disabled children did well from those on which they did poorly by using the Broverman and Klaiber distinction between perceptual-motor tasks and perceptual-restructuring tasks.[25] The reading-disabled children were strongest on tasks that required an holistic comprehension of relationships in information and use of this knowledge for meaningful manipulation of information. They were weakest on those subtests involving recall and fast rote processing of information.

In some of the studies reviewed by McLeod, the strengths of the reading-disabled children were so distinct that they constituted clear intellectual superiority. For example in a study by Harold Burks and Paul Bruce, a group of disabled readers were one and one-half years ahead of the national norms for their age in performance on the picture arrangement subtest.[26] They were nearly a full year ahead on the block design subtest, and about three-quarters of a year ahead on the picture completion and comprehension subtests. Considering that these represent averages for a whole group and that it is highly unlikely that all of the children followed this exact pattern, some of the children must have been quite gifted in their spatial ability.

It was on the basis of observed spatial ability strengths among learning-disabled children that Alexander Bannatyne came to speculate that there may be an inherited tendency for some people to possess a brain structure that is specialized for spatial competence. The evidence for Bannatyne's hypothesis is related to research on cerebral asymmetry. This research is reviewed in greater detail in Chapter 5. In simplist terms, the Bannatyne hypothesis goes something like this. Spatial thinking involves manipulative visualization. Visual processes require the two visual projection areas that are situated in the rear parts of both the left and right sides of our brains. Since the things that we see on the right side of us are received only by the projection area on the left side of our brains and the things we see on the left side are received only by that on the right side of our brains, full coordination of visualized thinking must require a careful coordination between information that is being processed in both sides of our brains.

> It is self-evident that the manipulation of objects in three-dimensional space very frequently requires the subject to work in two or three visual dimensions which will involve both his visual fields and very often both hands. The architect at his drawing board, the engineer, mechanic, surgeon, dentist, airline pilot, car driver, factory worker, farmer, research scientist, sculptor, artist and designer usually utilize both visual fields and both hands in their daily work. This bilateral visuo-spatial activity must involve both hemispheres simultaneously at the very least in the motor, haptic, kinesthetic and visual areas. . . . The alteration between the two may be rapid, or it may be dependent on the importance of the task being carried out in either visual field or by either hand; i.e., during which moment is the dentist manipulating the mirror with his left hand and the drill with his right? However, it is very likely that the two hemispheres act spatially in a fully integrated synthesis of simultaneous functioning in most visuo-spatial tasks.[27]

Bannatyne* speculates that such required coordination in visualized thinking may be in conflict with the fact that the left side of most people's brains is specialized for verbal processes. An either–or situation may arise in which a child is either specialized to emphasize the use of the left hemisphere for language skills or is specialized to emphasize the coordination between both sides of the brain in order to achieve more efficient spatial thinking. Since the right hemisphere is more heavily specialized for spatial thinking, Bannatyne suggests that in order to achieve the needed coordination between the two hemispheres, there must be some kind of executive control center for spatial thinking in the right hemisphere. When this spatial control center is rather dominant for all thinking, a child is competent in spatial ability but deficient in language ability. In the so-called "visuo-spatial brain, while language functioning remains relatively dominant in the left hemisphere . . . both hemispheres actively participate in all behaviors involving spatial tasks. . . . The left hemisphere language functions subserve the more dominant right hemisphere spatial functions."[28]

Bannatyne supports this speculation by pointing to two common observations about poor readers. First, they have a greater tendency than other children to be poorly lateralized, and second, they tend to experience left–right confusion. Poor lateralizaton can mean a number of things. By observing certain behaviors one can make assumptions about which side of the brain is most involved in controlling these behaviors. For example, if a child is observed as he eats, writes, or throws a ball, it can be seen which hand is used for each activity. If a child is asked to hop on one foot, which foot will he use? If a child is asked to make the shape of a telescope with his hands and then asked to look through the telescope, which eye will be used for sighting? The side of the brain opposite to the limb or eye that is being used in the activity tends to be most dominant in controlling the behavior. A more technical approach to studying lateralization would involve the use of the electroencephalogram (EEG). A certain type of brain wave pattern called the *alpha wave* indicates that the hemisphere of the brain from which it is received is at rest. By observing alpha wave patterns received from the left and right sides of the brain of a person who is carrying out various ac-

---

* From Alexander Bannatyne, *Language, Reading and Learning Disabilities*, 1971. Courtesy of Charles C Thomas, Publisher, Springfield, Ill.

tivities, one can make assumptions as to which side of the brain is more at rest and which is more active during each activity.

As a result of research on lateralization, it has been found that many poor readers are among those who are poorly lateralized. In some cases, this might mean that a child will tend to throw a ball with the right hand but hop on the left foot. In other cases, this might mean that when alpha waves are observed from children who are reading, there will be much less tendency among poor readers for only one side of the brain to be predominantly active. In other words, the poor readers are actively using both left and right cerebral hemispheres for reading rather than relying predominantly on their left verbal hemisphere. The neuropsychologists Hacaen and Ajuriaguerra conclude from their observations: "Our study (of laterality in poor readers) shows that the group of children with dyslexia is statistically different from the normal group when one considers the relative proportions of the lateral dominances, and that the children with dyslexia are not more often left-handed than the controls but more poorly lateralized. The high proportion of crossed dominance (ambidexterity) in the group of the youngest children with dyslexia is what appears to be most characteristic."[29]

The other observations on disabled readers is that, more than other children, they tend to experience left–right confusion. For example they might have difficulty recognizing the differences between a *b* and a *d*. The two letters are mirror images of each other. The tendency toward left–right confusion is, in a way, a natural, adaptive phenomenon. During the course of evolution, it was crucial that any animal learn to recognize that the lion who walks toward the left is the same lion who previously walked toward the right. Otherwise our animal ancestors would have always seen the same lion as being two different things, and not applied lessons learned from the left-facing lion to the right-facing lion. And there is evidence that as a result of this evolutionary necessity, our brains encode spatial information both as we see it and also in its left–right reversal.[30] This is a valuable adaptation in the world of objects. In nature, a lion is a lion, is a lion, whichever way he is facing. In reading, however, a *b* is not a *d*. To the extent that a child tends to treat letters as spatial objects rather than symbols, left–right confusions will be natural.

For Bannatyne, poor lateralization and left–right confusion are closely associated. Research tends to indicate that both often occur in the same reading-disabled children.[31] The thrust of Bannatyne's position seems to be that if both hemispheres are primarily serving spatial processes, then the left hemisphere will not be particularly proficient in carrying out its language functions. Reading and writing may be processed in a somewhat spatial manner on both sides of the brain. Also, the ability to make left–right distinctions, presumed to derive from left-hemisphere language specialization, is not highly developed. The child is programmed for visuo-spatial thinking but disabled in language. This is an interesting line of reasoning, which seems to relate in varying degrees with the assortment of facts that Bannatyne presents. It seems to fit with the observation that some people possessing exceptional spatial skills are ambidextrous.[32]

The difficulty with Bannatyne's speculations is that the underlying physiology reality is bound to be much more complex than his speculations. In spite of the fact that poor readers may share certain characteristics such as specialization for spatial skills, poor lateralization, and left–right confusion, there is no general tendency for people who experience poor lateralization and left–right confusion to be superior in spatial ability. So far, physiological research has not located any particular place in the right hemisphere that could be considered Bannatyne's "executive control center" for spatial thought processes. Physiological research has clearly not proceeded far enough to give a very clear picture of the way these variables relate to each other. More importantly, the research has not reached a point where it can accurately guide educational practice.

The more valuable aspect of Bannatyne's work are his observations on dyslexic children who possess considerable spatial ability. We should share with Bannatyne the urgency of locating these children and preventing them from being poorly understood and poorly served in educational institutions which seem to have little idea of their capabilities. Bannatyne said, "In my work, I have found boys in classes for mentally retarded children who, on tests, had a WISC verbal scale I.Q. of 75 points or less, and a spatial ability I.Q. (Picture Completion, plus Block Design, plus Object Assembly) of which any professional engineer or architect would have been proud. One boy had a spatial ability I.Q. of 145 — he was described by his teachers in that most condescending of phrases as being clever with his hands."[33]

When a dyslexic child is truly exceptional in the extent of his spatial ability, he often survives the mistreatment to find an appropriate place for himself in the world. But the misery the child may suffer while trying to conform to verbosely dominated schools can only be imagined by those who have themselves suffered the "Alice in Wonderland" experience, the experience of being in a place where nothing can quite be put together to make sense. In this confusing out-of-place world, the child has difficulty performing to control his destiny, and then is punished by low grades or failure for the fact that he is out of place. And this occurs in spite of the fact that the child can perform many important tasks with excellence.

> Most genetic dyslexic boys go into trades and professions which utilize their visuo-spatial skills, becoming designers, mechanics, engineers, farmers, surgeons, dentists, architects, drivers, pilots, artists and sculptors. . . . Many of them have university degrees and all tell the same tale, which always includes several of the following characteristics: somewhat slow speech development in early childhood, difficulty with auditory sequencing, closure and blending, difficulty in learning to read initially and a residual problem in spelling which usually persists into adulthood. Most of these men have clear, logical, scientific minds which can create, plan, organize and develop visuo-spatial materials and processes in a highly competent way. . . . They can also handle absolute symbols, such as those used in chemistry, and are very able to cope with abstract reasoning. One person, for example, is a professor of physics who did not learn to speak until he was three or read until he was eight. However, in spite of this slow start, he became an excellent scientist in school and today is a highly original and excellent physicist.[34]

These cases are the fortunate ones. But it is unlikely that most children who are misunderstood as children go this far with their talents. The fact that the average school has little understanding or appreciation for this type of child has got to be one of the greatest sources of wasted human talent in our society.

REFERENCES

1. Galton, F. *Inquiries into Human Faculty and Its Development*. London: Dent, 1973, p. 58.
2. *Ibid.*, pp. 58-59.
3. *Ibid.*, p. 59.
4. *Ibid.*, p. 61.
5. Einstein, A. Letter to Jacques Hadamard. In *The Creatve Process* by Brewster

Ghiselin. New York: Mentor Books, 1952, p. 43.

6. Roe, A. A study of imagery in research scientists. *Journal of Personality, 19*:464, 1950-1951.

7. *Ibid.*, p. 463.

8. Bartlett, F.C. *Remembering.* Cambridge, Mass.: Harvard University Press, 1932.

9. Kuhlman, C.K. *Visual Imagery in Children.* Ph.D. thesis, Harvard University, 1960.

10. Mallory, W.A. Abilities and developmental changes in elaborative strategies in paired-associate learning of young children. *Journal of Educational Psychology, 63*:202-217, 1972; Das, J.P. Structure of cognitive abilities. *Journal of Educational Psychology, 65*:103-108, 1973; Levin, J.R., Divine-Hawkins, P., Kerst, S.M., and Guttman, J. Individual differences in learning from pictures and words. *Journal of Educational Psychology, 66*:296-303, 1974; Labouvie-Vief, G., Levin, J.R., and Urberg, K.A. The relationship between selected cognitive abilities and learning. *Journal of Educational Psychology, 67*:558-569, 1975.

11. MacLeod, C.M., Hunt, E.B., and Mathews, N.N. Individual differences in the verification of sentence-picture relationships. *Journal of Verbal Learning and Verbal Behavior, 17*:493-507, 1978; Sternberg, R.J., and Weil, E.M. An aptitude x strategy interaction in linear syllogistic reasoning. *Journal of Educational Psychology, 72*:226-239, 1980.

12. Koussy, A. The visual perception of space. *British Journal of Psychology,* Monograph Supplement, No. 20, 1935.

13. Clarke, G. *The Range and Nature of Factors in Perceptual Tests.* Ph.D. thesis, University of London, 1936.

14. Emmett, W.G. Evidence for a space factor at 11 plus and earlier. *British Journal of Psychology, 2*:3-16, 1949; Stephenson, W. Tetrad-differences for non-verbal sub-tests. *British Journal of Psychology, 22*:167-185, 1931; Smith, I.M. *An Investigation into the Problem of Measuring Spatial Ability in Pupils of 11 or 12.* Ph.D. thesis, University of Manchester, 1952; Drew, L.J. *An Experimental Enquiry into the Methods of Selection for Technical Education Based on Multiple Factor-Analysis.* M.Ed. thesis, University of Leeds, 1944.

15. Smith, I.M. *Spatial Ability: Its Educational and Social Significance.* London: University of London Press, 1964, p. 53.

16. Broverman, D.M., and Klaiber, E.L. Negative relationships between abilities. *Psychometrika, 34*:5, 1969.

17. *Ibid.*, pp. 5-18.

18. Smith, 1964, *op. cit.*, pp. 321-351.

19. Yates, A., and Barr, F. Selection for secondary technical courses. *Educational Research, 2*:143-148, 1960.

20. Nisbet, J., and Buchan, J. The long-term follow-up of assessments at age eleven. *British Journal of Educational Psychology, 29*:1-8, 1959.

21. Smith, 1964, *op. cit.*, p. 31.

22. Broverman and Klaiber, *op. cit.*, p. 5-18.

23. Keyes, S. *Biological and Social Factors in the Development of Spatial Ability.* Thesis prospectus, Harvard University, 1977.

24. McLeod, J. A comparison of WISC sub-test scores of preadolescent successful and unsuccessful readers. *Australian Journal of Psychology, 17*:220-228, 1965.
25. Broverman and Klaiber, *op. cit.,* p. 6.
26. Burks, H.F., and Bruce, P. The characteristics of poor and good readers as disclosed by the WISC. *Journal of Educational Psychology, 46*:448-493, 1955.
27. Bannatyne, A. *Language, Reading and Learning Disabilities.* Springfield, Ill.: Charles C Thomas, Publisher, 1971, p. 218.
28. *Ibid.,* p. 225.
29. Hecaen, H., and Ajuriaguerra, J. *Left-Handedness.* New York: Grune and Stratton, 1964.
30. Corballis, M.C., and Beale, I.L. *The Psychology of Left and Right.* New York: John Wiley and Sons, 1976.
31. Harris, A.J. Lateral dominance, directional confusion, and reading disability. *Journal of Psychology, 44*:283-294, 1957.
32. Burt, C. *The Backward Child.* London: University of London Press, 1950.
33. Bannatyne, *op. cit.,* p. 378.
34. Bannatyne, *op. cit.,* p. 379.

Chapter 4

BIOGRAPHY

REUBEN

REUBEN was fascinating to me from the first time that I met him. He was very pleasant in attitude, and when he came in the door, he would respond to greetings with a friendly "hi." Otherwise, words were used with exceptional frugality, and mostly to request paper, pens, and magic markers for doing his drawing. He would draw for hours, making technically impressive sketches of racing cars with all of the elaborate, imaginative details that only a preadolescent boy can fully appreciate. Reuben could get his friends to participate in the drawing for a time, but he was always the one to start the drawing, and he carried on long after the others had had their fill.

The skill of the drawings indicated unusual ability for an eight-year-old; this, combined with Reuben's nonverbal tendencies, indicated that Reuben might have a specialized strength for spatial skills. Formal confirmation of this came a few months later. In order to get a clear picture of the variations in Reuben's skill patterns, he was tested with the WISC-R. As one might easily have guessed, his block-design score, the most spatial test in the battery, indicated a very exceptional level of ability. His performance on the spatial, conceptual, and reasoning parts of the test resulted in a composite score that could be considered at a gifted level in spite of the fact that two of the subtest scores, coding and digit span, were slightly below average, which is a classic pattern.

When I talked to Reuben's parents about his development, the tension of years of uneasiness was immediately evident. The fact that a child could be considered gifted in a specialized way may provide some relief from concern about slow development in school-related skills, but a child still has to live in a world where reading and writing are among the conventional expectations. Concerned parents won't just ignore this even when they are trying to be patient

76

— a patience that for them has gone on for several years.

Reuben had had an initial start with speaking when he was about thirteen months old. He picked up a few words such as *no, mama, dada,* and *tra* for truck. But then much of this initial development went away, and acquisition of further speaking skills didn't start again until Reuben was nearly three. During this time, *tra* was a favorite word applied to anything that impressed Reuben. As months went by with no words added to his vocabulary, the concern of his parents grew. His mother, a professional writer, kept a record of this development: "There was a long time when he said 'tra' most of the time. I just couldn't understand why. He was a big kid. He was thriving physically. He was walking. He was an early walker. All his friends were quite verbal. He played with his friends. He didn't speak, but he didn't need to."[1]

Reuben got along well with other children, had many friends, and was a favorite play companion for many of them. It was clear that the lack of speech did not include withdrawal from other people. If anything, the opposite was true. It was as if his other interests, his capabilities, compensated for his lack of speech, and other children would seek him out for the fun they could find with him. It was as if they could play together and a commonly understood nonverbal code could guide their interactions and expectations without the necessity of speech. While Reuben wasn't getting speech together himself, he was understanding speech very well. His mother carried out elaborate tests of this. She reported, "I would give him problems. I would build barricades for him when he was first starting to walk, and make him go around them to fetch things. I would ask him to go get one thing, then two or three things two rooms away. He did very well. He always did well. That's why we were not too alarmed."

Finally, at age three, Reuben, began again to add vocabulary to his speech, and to put sentences together; however, even that was a slow development. When he entered school at age five, Reuben could use speech to describe situations with some complexity, but it was rare that he would make the effort, and it took time for him to construct his sentences. "Never said much," his father observed, "and any time he did it was a wrenching kind of experience. You could see the effort that it took. And if you didn't have a lot of time to wait, it was trying."

Sometimes it would seem as if the thoughts he was attempting to convey were somewhat more complex than the meaning load of the sentences Reuben could readily construct, and Reuben would get lost in the difficulties. "He could," his mother said, "stop right in the middle and try to figure out what he wants to say, and lose you completely, or else go off on some tangent."

The fact that his awareness was running far beyond the capacities of his language use was clear from the extent of his preverbal memory. The events of his earlier years were clear in his mind in considerable detail even when he had never spoken of the details before. The details were evidently recorded in some imagery that he was able to retrieve with ease at a much later time and then describe to others in verbal terms. The extent of this ability was so fascinating to his parents that his mother went to some effort to check the accuracy of what Reuben was recalling. She said, "When he did start to talk when he was about three, he remembered things that happened when he was about one. Who brought him things. He remembered the situation, the person, things I'd forgotten. I write a lot so I had my journals to go back and check. And he was right."

During the preverbal period, when his parents were wondering if Reuben would ever get speech together, they were also seeing the potential for precociousness in the way Reuben could manipulate objects and carry out his drawings. Around age one and one-half, Reuben was playing with a building kit called Fisher Technic®. The fitting together of the parts of this kit can be challenging to many adults. Reuben seemed to readily comprehend the problems involved and to construct with ease. More recently he was given one of the most complicated Lego® sets made. Reuben immediately went to the most complicated example given in the instructions and just built it. It had an engine with moving pistons.

Reuben's father is an architect and has taken an interest in Reuben's drawings. Sometimes his father will suggest drawing problems having to do with things like perspective or motion so that Reuben can work out his own solutions. "I might say, 'hey, you know, if that car were driving away from you, it would look an awful lot different than the way you're drawing it. You would see part of the back end, and the side. You would see part of the roof.' Within five minutes he's drawing beautifully in perspective."

Reuben loves to construct things whether it is model cars and airplanes or play houses and forts. There are times when he would build all day if not interrupted. His drawing is often a way of communicating ideas or telling a story. Reuben's father describes this: "Drawings are always story telling. His sister might make up a story to go along with the drawing; Reuben has the story in the drawing. She might draw a picture of a little girl and say, 'This is a little girl picking a flower in the sun whose mother just called her.' Reuben will draw the mother calling the little girl who's picking the flower with the sun out."

Reuben's parents describe his memory as being quite outstanding in a certain way. This might appear to be different from the pattern of the spatially specialized child, except that Reuben's memory strengths seem to be of a very special kind. He remembers events from the preverbal period with great clarity, and in exact sequence; however, the memory is being derived from visual and sensory imagery, and not from a verbal coding. His mother assumes that "there has to be a lot of imagery because it's hard for him to verbalize it. It's like he knows it in his mind, but he doesn't know the words to tell it. It comes in a halting way." With Reuben, the direct evidence of not being able to associate words with events and objects is not always there because he tends not to ask for help. He doesn't say, "What was that thing?" or "Who was that person?" Rather, Reuben may stop in the middle of a sentence and wait until he comes up with the word, or he might simply discontinue the conversation. "Sometimes he stops short of informing you," his mother said, "that it's a word that's missing and not a whole idea, or that he completely forgot about it."

His specialized memory extends to sound patterns. In one sense, this makes Reuben good at spelling. If spelling is approached as a whole pattern that he can put together in a start-to-finish sequence, Reuben is very good. Phonetic spelling, however, is difficult for him, and if he gets stopped in the middle of a word, he must usually start over to get it right. One might assume that the memory code takes a form similar to a visual image, that it depends on the holistic sense. The pattern as a whole is the thing that is coded, and the separate bits cannot be dealt with very successfully outside of the pattern. This fits with the observations of Fadely and Hosler and their recommendation of using this holistic sense as the basis for teaching spelling.[2]

Reuben enjoys music, especially the popular music he hears on television. He takes cello lessons. He does fairly well at learning songs and scales, especially when these are dealt with as start-to-finish patterns. Reuben is learning to read music notes in terms of going from notation to playing, but he has more difficulty applying the correct verbal names to the notes he is playing.

Although Reuben has many friends, and is a favorite playmate for other children because of the nifty spatial-mechanical things he can do, on more superficial grounds he might be seen as quiet and reserved. Reuben attends a small school where sharing meetings are a part of the daily routine. In the four years he has attended the school, he has rarely spoken out in meetings. "There were times," Reuben's mother said, "when we would go to a party and take him with us. He would sit on the couch and not make a sound — watching people, trying to drink in the scene. Gradually, he would start to feel comfortable or less noticed himself, and he would go into doing something."

Reuben has been slow to learn reading and writing skills, but with the tutoring he is now receiving, he is improving quickly. He is an intellectually capable child with a growing sense of humor and a growing ability to communicate his ideas to others. For Reuben, getting the kind of intellectual stimulation he needs can be a problem. His lack of verbal response to teachers can leave them without the kind of feedback they usually look for to confirm learning. He will need those situations where his form of constructing, experimenting, and expressing are recognized and guided toward higher levels of accomplishment.

NILDA

As a part of conducting a research project on bilingual education programs, for nearly a year, I spent a good portion of my time doing observations of children in bilingual classrooms.[3] That's where I met Nilda. Nilda has an Irish last name and is a red-haired, green-eyed, freckle-faced girl one might expect to meet in Dublin, except at the time I met her, Nilda spoke only Spanish. Her family had come straight from Puerto Rico only the year before. Initially, Nilda was most interesting to me because she had a creative way of sitting. Rules were fairly strict in her classroom. Nilda had to spend most of her time at her school desk. But for a girl who found such constraint to be unacceptable, and who had an imaginative mind, even a rigid school chair presented many possibilities. One might say without exaggeration that all the infinite possible sitting postures were tried at one time or another, and most of them in quick succession during the course of each school day, including the head draped backward over the front of the desk and one leg over the backrest. Nilda's teacher tried as she might to restrict this dynamic posturing, but eventually arrived at a wise sense that the need for it came from some drive deep in Nilda's nature. The teacher learned to work around it by having Nilda sit in a place where she would be minimally disturbing to other children.

Nilda was bright and responsive about things that interested her, but her reading, writing, and arithmetic suffered. She enjoyed arts and crafts, and her work became much more focused when it involved art projects. Even more than arts and crafts, Nilda loved dancing. The teacher had organized a dance pageant as a part of getting recognition for the bilingual program, and Nilda enjoyed this activity thoroughly. For most of the other children, the pageant was a social event that made school more interesting. For Nilda, it was something she threw herself into with complete energy and flair. The folk dance format of the event was limited in its creative possibilities, but the teacher recognized Nilda's joy for the dancing and arranged for Nilda and a small group of other children to do a special dance which allowed more expression.

I was convinced there was something special about Nilda from these initial observations, but two years later my interest was again raised when Nilda took a figural test of creativity. This is a test in which the creative potential of children is assessed through the pictures they draw. Nilda's score on the test was about as high as can be achieved — easily at the ninety-ninth percentile. This score might have qualified her for the program for gifted students, except that her academic skills were below average, and it was thought that she would find it difficult relating to more academically inclined children. Following up on Nilda's love for dancing seemed to make more sense, and arrangements were made for her to attend a creative dance program.

In the dance program, students were taught elements of dance movement and then encouraged to fit these elements together in unique ways. Nilda took to this right away, especially the unique side of it. Other students accepted many of the obvious possibilities in putting together the dance elements. Nilda often improvised her own elements and put them together in a dynamic, flowing way, which marked her as special, even in a school for those who were special. Today, Nilda is a high school senior. She is still dancing; now with a semiprofessional company, and showing considerable promise.

But what of the academics that Nilda could never quite focus on when I first saw her in third grade? Nilda has never adapted very well to her schoolwork. She managed to get by until she was a freshman in high school. The poor work and poor attendance were too much, and she failed two subjects. There were other failures. With makeup work in summer school, she managed to stay only half a year behind her class. She will graduate in due time, but with a sense that schoolwork was a miserable diversion from her real interests. Most of Nilda's teachers are quite understanding of her dilemma, and some have pushed things pretty far in finding ways for Nilda to get by. But no matter how strongly Nilda may feel the necessity for approaching life the way she does, one also gets the sense that she feels that she has failed, that she has let other people down, especially her parents.

Nilda's parents have been concerned about her schoolwork from the time she started school. They correctly insist that Nilda is very bright, and they have always been determined that she should perform well in school. After Nilda failed the two freshman-year subjects, her parents insisted that she not study dance for a year. Nilda's studies improved a little during this time, but when she was allowed to return to dancing, it seemed to be an admission that dancing was the only thing Nilda enjoyed rather than a reward to Nilda for being a better scholar. The back-and-forth tension between Nilda's natural feeling for dance and her parent's insistance that she should be a better student has gone on for years. Even now that Nilda is near completing high school, her parents are still looking for some way to rectify the situation. They want her to attend a special summer school. Knowing that Nilda will need a way to make a living, they would also like her to study accounting, and Nilda reluctantly accepts the logic of her parents' thinking.

This kind of tension is common among children whose giftedness diverges from school-related areas. Since school is the primary source of recognition and evaluation for a young person, considerable confusion may develop. The child often gets some recognition for unusual talent, but at the same time is constantly being told of inadequacies in schoolwork. There may be a feeling of pride over accomplishments. But this is outweighed by a general feeling of inadequacy, which persists in spite of the accomplishments. When I talked to Nilda about the variations in her performance, it seemed this was such a problem to her that she could hardly sort things out enough to talk in an openly assertive way about it, even though her behavior in succeeding at some things, but failing at others, has been abundantly assertive in its consequences for years. It was as if she was accepting the idea that she should want to be an accountant as her parents wish, even though she has never taken a single step in that direction. It is as if she accepts the idea that she should have been a better student and judges herself, as her parents do, accordingly.

Her parents have the same ambivalence about dance. In her younger years, when others were beginning to recognize Nilda's potential, her parents often avoided participating in this recognition as if doing so might detract from their insistence that Nilda become a good student. When Nilda eventually won an award for her dance, the trophy was given a prominent place in the living room; Nilda's father framed the newspaper report of the award and hung it on the wall. Yet, one gets a feeling that her parents would gladly trade any dance award for twelve years of even slightly above-average performance in school.

This kind of experience is so common for some types of gifted children that it should be considered one of the major unsolved problems in the field. It would not be fair to suggest that the concern of parents and teachers about the poor academic performance of some gifted children is not justified. Yet, biography on genius indicates that poor academic performance can often be irrelevant to outstanding performance in certain fields. Although we should never deliberately undermine the school performance of any child on the grounds that giftedness makes it irrelevant, it sometimes becomes obvious that higher levels of academic achievement will never be an ingredient of the performance of some gifted children. When that happens, the child and all those concerned must be helped to understand the direction the child is going. Parents must be encouraged to give their children a sense of accomplishment, rather than conflict about their genius.

MARY LAYCOCK

To see her at work, to watch this sixty-seven-year-old California woman running an active teacher workshop, selling ideas for bettering mathematics education, one wouldn't suspect that when she was very young, doctors never expected her to live to adulthood. At age six, she weighed 25 pounds, and she was so frail that her parents couldn't allow her to go to school until she was nine. One would hardly guess it because Mary Laycock is one of this country's most energetic and successful educational innovators. She teaches mathematics to gifted children at the Nueva School and Learning Center in Hillsborough, California, publishes books on mathematics education, and consults with schools and educational agencies throughout the United States and the world. During her years as an educator, Mary has taken on the mission of finding methods of teaching mathematics in such a way that the basic structure can be understood, not just memorized. Much of this effort has involved developing ideas for representing concepts through manipulative materials.

Although Mary Laycock's ideas have not been developed exclusively for the benefit of children whose thought processes run in a spatial direction, they nevertheless are so firmly grounded in spatial concepts that they are ideally suited for use with spatial children. The fitting of her ideas to the unique needs of spatial children probably started with experiences early in her teaching career. As a math teacher in the Oak Ridge schools in Tennessee, she found that counselors began to identify children who had high IQs but low achievement and began to assign them her classes. The counselors recognized that she was doing something special for these children. Mary Laycock said the following regarding this experience: "Then I did not know why I was so successful in interesting and exciting them in mathematics. We built models and projects for everything. The cases were full; we carried them to show at the math conferences."[4]

It was certainly no accident that Mary Laycock's career went in this direction. She is, herself, primarily a spatial thinker. She was fortunate to grow up in a very literate family; this helped her to develop reading at an early age so that she never experienced any language-related difficulties. Her father was a humanistically inclined clergyman who read extensively and encouraged scholarship as a virtue. "His theme was that only how much you used your mind and were considerate to others were you of value." Her language development was, ironically, helped by the frailty of her youth. Her mother taught her to read and write, and the encouragement of her family led to rapid educational development. When she finally went to school, she became an excellent student, especially in mathematics. Her seventh grade teacher made a special effort to teach her algebra because Mary's family was moving to Mobile, Alabama, the next year; it was thought that Mary was advanced enough to go directly to high school in Mobile. In Mobile, Mary graduated as valedictorian of a large high school class.

Yet, throughout this story of unusual achievement, there were aspects of learning that were not so easy. Because of the academic encouragement of her family, she studied Latin for seven years; however, it was a struggle. She said, "How I slaved! Language . . . even English, especially spelling, required an enormous amount of time to master." She read well but somewhat slowly. "I did not like tests that were related to speed," Mary said. Memorizing details was always a problem. This could have caused difficulties in geometry where formal proofs can be tedious in detail, except that she was so good at making up her own proofs. She said, "The teacher encouraged this and almost always had me share the proof I had written, as well as the one in the book that the other kids memorized."

Graphic arts were an important preoccupation for her father, but Mary didn't take an interest in this as a child. It sometimes seemed to her that graphic arts were a distraction from other important things. "My daddy was a painter and potter and would get so lost in his hobby that as a teen-ager I felt he neglected earning a living to pursue his art." But Mary did enjoy making three-dimensional structures out of paper. The geometric approach to understanding was what suited her best. In college, she would work on mathematics with her best friend. Mary would work out problems geometrically, her friend algebraically. "When we got the same answer we knew we were correct."

Mary describes her thought processes as being primarily spatial in nature. She likes to get a feeling for the whole picture, or the systematic qualities of a subject; then the details fall in place easily. She enjoys drawing and making things. She understands things better if they are demonstrated rather than talked about, and in her training workshops for teachers, she insists on showing how her materials work with hands-on experience for the participants. Mary is most comfortable with creative approaches to learning. She said, "I tell children there are always ways to solve a problem . . . . I question everything I hear or read!!! I often improvise to get a job done . . . in fact I like that style. I like problems with a twist . . . . For years I have had students that could pick the answer out of the air but could not explain how they got it. I tell them to rejoice and help them work backward to prove it. I think they are the truly gifted kind."

But then there are the memory problems that plague many spatial thinkers. Mary has trouble remembering disconnected, detailed information. She stated, "Names are my downfall! I can tell how well a person understands me but have real trouble remembering the name." Mary has developed strategies for remembering things by hanging details together in her mental imagery. She has also learned to make lists to prod herself on what must come next.

There were eight years of piano lessons that Mary struggled through as a child, but she confesses to have no special appreciation for music. At age nine, she had lessons from the theory teacher at the University of Kansas. "She taught me all the music theory that she was teaching her college freshmen; I made the highest grade on their mid-term. I loved it! There was so much order and pattern in it." The beauty of the order was more attractive than the music itself.

As a successful educational innovator, today she feels no uneasiness about relating to other people, especially when it involves professional interests and concerns. She does, nevertheless, identify with the common experiences of childhood shyness. Mary remembers herself as being quiet, reserved, and serious. She feared large group situations, and to make a formal presentation in front of other people required much effort. Today she is, of course, no longer stagestruck when presenting to groups of strangers, but still doesn't enjoy superficial social gatherings. Getting together with professional friends and colleagues is most enjoyable. For doing her work, privacy is sometimes needed. "After my husband goes to bed, I read or write on my word processor, or build a model for the children or for myself."

Today, one of the focuses of Mary's efforts is the publishing business she runs with her husband. In 1971, when her most extensive manuscript was ready for publication, no publisher would consider it because it recommended the use of materials from a wide variety of other publishers.[5] Not wanting to lose the integrity of the book, her husband decided they would publish it themselves. "My husband said I had seen him lose money on the stock market and had never complained. . . . We would publish ourselves." Within a year, the book had sold in every state and in seven foreign countries. At present, they publish about seventy-five different manuscripts.

Mary has a passion for improving the methods by which children are taught elementary mathematics. "The real problem," she said, "is to get some real mathematics into the understanding of the elementary teacher who only knows the final short cut algorithms of arithmetic." Her success in this task will most certainly lead to benefits for other spatial children.

PABLO RUIZ PICASSO

Pablo Picasso was born on October 25, 1881, in Malaga on the southern coast of Spain. For a child with Picasso's natural talents, it was most fortunate that his father was an artist. His father never became well known for his own artwork; however, he was an academically trained painter, a teacher of art, the curator of an art museum, and the friend of many accomplished artists. This was just the right setting for the spawning of genius. But the contribution of Picasso's father went much further than providing the perfect setting. The father understood his son's needs and weaknesses as few parents do. With a perfect understanding of the possibilities and the needed ingredients for development, he protected and guided an otherwise vulnerable child.

Picasso's inclination toward artistry was seen from early childhood. There is a legend that his first spoken word was *piz, piz,* the baby form of *lapiz* or pencil. Evidently, even when he was first learning to speak, he had an inclination to draw. Picasso's natural grasp of the structure of drawing was amazing to those around him. A popular game among the children of Malaga was the tracing of arabesque patterns in the dirt. These are the designs that the Moors brought to Spain from North Africa and incorporated into their buildings. Part of the game was to start at any point in the pattern and to have such an accurate understanding of all relationships in the pattern that a perfect rendering could be achieved. No one surpassed Pablo Picasso at this game. The skill became a characteristic of his artwork. "As a very old man in years he would still start a drawing anywhere at all, just as he had done when he was a little boy, amazing his cousins Concha and Maria by beginning a dog or a cock at any point they chose to name — the claws, the tail — or by cutting the forms out of paper with his aunt's embroidery scissors on the same terms."[6]

The young Picasso would spend much of his time in school drawing. He must have been so astonishingly noticeable for his talent that his teachers allowed him to carry on to an extent that would have led any other student to receive a beating.

> Even in a very easy-going establishment a child who sat, not minding his book but drawing bulls or the live pigeon he had brought in his bosom, and who got up without leave to gape out of the window, would have been sharply rebuked at the least and more probably flogged; but not Picasso. . . . It does not appear that he was a wicked, turbulent, or dissipated pupil, but rather that he belonged on another plane: the master and even more surprisingly the other boys accepted this and they neither complained nor imitated his example when he stood up and walked out of the room altogether, looking for the headmaster's wife, to whom he was much attached. "I used to follow her about like a puppy," he said.[7]

Actually, the tolerance of Picasso's behavior derived as much from a recognition of the hopelessness of his academic skills as from an appreciation for his artistry. He was an exceptionally dull student who had difficulties learning to read, to write, and to do arithmetic. Throughout his life, he was never at home with the alphabet. His approach to spelling seemed to be pretty much his own. He eventually learned to do calculations well enough to be a shrewd businessman. But this was not true when he was a child. Learning to count was difficult. Telling time was always a problem. A story is told of how an uncle one day passed by the school. Picasso, being particularly anxious about having to stay at school, called out for his uncle to take him away. His uncle asked when school would be let out. Picasso replied, "At one," thinking that because one is the first number it would also come first.[8]

For a child so naturally capable in drawing it might seem strange that he had difficulty with the shape of letters. Whatever the attraction of his artwork, his handwriting was messy. In line with Bannatyne's speculations about the spatially competent brain, it is of particular interest that Picasso had difficulty with mirror reversals and left-right confusion.[9] "His mirror-version of the final question-mark . . . He sometimes inverted the esses of his signature, and when he took to etching and engraving he could not or would not grasp that the printing of the plate necessarily reversed the legend. It is as though there were some confusion in the mental process that separates right from left."[10]

Fortunately, the primary reaction to Picasso's academic in-competence was tolerance. This was invaluable to a person so specialized in ability, and represented an unusual degree of enlightenment. Some of the tolerance may have derived from respect for a budding genius, but more likely it derived from a recognition of his hopeless incompetence for academic work. Picasso first attended a parochial school but was soon switched to a private school after he suffered some illness and was declared a "delicate child." The illness may well have been brought on by the stress of attending a parochial school where the demands were beyond his capability. In the private school, Picasso's puppy-like relationship to the headmaster's wife suggests that he was seen as defective for normal academic work. Picasso's constitutional infirmity perhaps was recognized from birth when he appeared to be stillborn but was brought to life by the resusitation of his uncle, the attending physician.

Picasso's nearly nonexistent performance in school was of little concern to his family until he was ten and they were preparing to move to LaCoruna in the northern part of Spain. In Malaga, he was under the protection of an extended and established middle-class family. His father began to wonder what would happen to his son in a strange city. In order to enter any school, Picasso would either have to pass an entrance examination or present a certificate of com-petence. The story is told that the father found a sympathetic friend who had the power to give a certificate. Picasso was taken to the friend for testing. To start the test, a simple addition problem was given. Picasso's first attempt to add the numbers was unsuccessful. A second chance was given. Picasso noticed that the examiner wrote the answer on a sheet of paper left deliberately where Picasso could see it. He copied the answer and thereupon received the only educa-tional certificate he was ever to be granted.

The relationship of father to son in this story is unique. The father taught Picasso the artistic techniques in vogue at the time.

The realistic, representational art that was standard in Spain had well-defined technical principles. These were commonly passed from one generation to the next without deviation. Although Picasso would break radically from this tradition soon after leaving Spain, the early training under the watchful eyes of his father provided a technical foundation to Picasso's work, which served him well throughout his life, even as he applied the techniques to a very different style of art.

Picasso's earliest preserved piece of work is an oil painting, which is thought to have been done when he was nine or ten years old. It is of a picador sitting on a horse in a bull ring. This painting is interesting because it provides an insight into the things that he observed in the world around him. It may also give a hint of feeling for the puny, blindfolded horse. Picasso probably saw many horses disemboweled in the bullring.[11]

Picasso's father played a unique role in the development of his genius. The genius was respected. This allowed the child to feel that it was his genius that counted, not that of the teacher. The father taught the son what he could, but then saw the limits of the teaching. Among the legends of Picasso's childhood, we are told that when his father recognized that he could teach him nothing more, he gave his brushes to Picasso and never painted again.[12] Whether this is taken to be a literal or fanciful report, it conveys the reality of the father's recognition of a superior talent.

ALBERT EINSTEIN

Albert Einstein was born in Ulm, Germany, in March 1879. As with Picasso, there is evidence of early precociousness and family encouragement for the field of study he would enter, although the evidence is not quite so striking. Einstein's family was involved in scientific professions. His father and his uncle Jacob carried on an electrical business of one kind or another throughout Einstein's childhood. Einstein remembered being shown a compass by his father around age five and being immediately impressed by such a simple instrument that revealed the implication of the force fields extending throughout space, which was supposed to be empty. The young Einstein was also amused by Uncle Jacob's personalized approach to alegebra. "Algebra is a merry science. We go hunting for a little animal whose name we don't know, so we call it X. When we bag our game, we pounce on it and give it its right name."[13]

Another Uncle, Casar, gave Einstein a model steam engine that impressed him so much that thirty years later Einstein would draw a sketch of it from memory.[14] The most significant influence on his developing mind probably came when Albert was about eleven. Max Talmey, a young medical student, became a frequent visitor of the Einstein household. Talmey took a special interest in Einstein because of the ease with which Einstein seemed to deal with abstract ideas in physics. Years later, Talmey reported, "He showed a particular inclination toward physics and took great pleasure in conversing on physical phenomena. I gave him therefore as reading matter . . . two works that were then quite popular in Germany. The boy was profoundly impressed by them."[15]

Later, Einstein developed a strong interest in mathematics, especially geometry, and Talmey brought more books. Before long, the abstractness of Albert's understanding moved beyond a point where Talmey could help.

> After a short time, a few months, he had worked through the whole book of Spieker. He thereupon devoted himself to higher mathematics, studying all by himself Luben's excellent works on the subject. . . . Soon the flight of his mathematical genius was so high that I could no longer follow. Thereafter philosophy was often a subject of our conversations. I recommended to him the reading of Kant. At that time he was still a child, only thirteen years old, yet Kant's works, incomprehensible to ordinary mortals, seemed to be clear to him.[16]

Around age sixteen, after his family had moved to Milan, Italy, Einstein wrote an essay outlining a possible line of investigation. This essay may represent the initial stages of reasoning that eventually led to the general theory of relativity, the most profound work of Einstein's life. The essay was sent to his Uncle Casar. Scientific interests may have provided a common mode of communication for the boy and his uncle, but Einstein seemed to recognize that sending a scientific essay to a family member might be seen as unusual. In the letter Einstein used his lack of correspondence as an excuse for sending the essay.

> I am really very happy that you are still interested in the little things I am doing and working on, even though we could not see each other for a long time, and I am such a terribly lazy correspondent. And yet I always hesitated to send you this (attached) note because it deals with a very

special topic; and besides, it is still rather naive and imperfect, as is to be expected from a young fellow like myself. I shall not mind it at all if you don't read this stuff; but you must recognize it at least as a modest attempt to overcome the laziness in writing which I have inherited from both of my dear parents.[17]

Einstein was beginning to delve into creatively profound ideas. Because he was not yet in a school or in an occupation where these ideas could be shared, he needed any kind of outlet he could find. There is more than a little loneliness in the lives of budding geniuses. Having no colleagues who are capable of fully appreciating their ideas, they sometimes unburden themselves on anyone willing to listen to ideas, which, to ordinary people, can seem like fantastic garbage. In his essay, Einstein described a course of research that could illuminate the nature of magnetism. He suggested that magnetism could come to be better understood "by measuring the elastic deformations and the acting deforming forces."[18] These ideas remained in the back of his mind until, nearly a decade later, they began to bear fruit.

Could a child with such obvious signs of developing genius show, at the same time, signs of intellectual difficulty? Indeed! In spite of Albert Einstein's international reputation as, perhaps, the genius of all time, as an adult, he was somewhat reluctant to speak about his difficulties in school as a child. This is often true of people who were taught to have doubts about themselves as children. The bitterness and embarrassment, no matter how trivial from an objective point of view, remain embedded in deeply hurting areas of consciousness and can never be easily related to others without emotion.

Biographers have had to piece together the bits of available information to arrive at speculations about his difficulties. The folk tales of Albert Einstein flunking his first year of algebra may not be entirely accurate, but they are not far from the truth. Einstein was a student whom teachers saw as having very poor prospects. There was a story in the family that when Hermann Einstein, Albert's father, asked the school headmaster "what profession his son should adopt, the answer was simply: It doesn't matter; he'll never make a success of anything."[19]

From the beginning, Einstein was maladapted to school. He was shy and withdrawn and was sometimes a troublemaker. Because he had shown some precocity for physical science and mathematics, he persevered in school up to age thirteen. Then, in spite of the hopes of his family that he would complete high school and go on to university study, he managed to get himself expelled from school. Young Einstein was notified that his "presence in the class is disruptive and affects the other students."[20]

The tone of this notification suggests that the reason for expulsion was behavioral. A tendency toward mischief can be its own reason for trouble, but behavioral problems often have their source in other maladaptive circumstances. If so, what might these circumstances have been in Einstein's case? Young Einstein was noted for his nonverbal nature. He had difficulty learning to speak. "One feature of his childhood about which there appears no doubt is the lateness with which he learned to speak. Even at the age of nine he was not fluent, while reminiscences of his youth stress hesitancies and the fact that he would reply to questions only after consideration and reflection. His parents feared he might be subnormal."[21] Although the details are not so clear, he also had some difficulty learning to read. A safe hunch is that he did not adapt well to the emphasis on verbal learning, which prevails in elementary school. Some formal language difficulty prevailed throughout his life. On a document as important as his doctoral dissertation, one would think a supreme effort would have been made to conform to scholarly expectations. Nonetheless, approval of the dissertation was much in doubt, and, in the words of one of his professors, could only be done by overlooking "crudeness in style and slips of the pen in formulas."[22]

Spatial imagery formed the most fundamental basis for his thought processes. After Einstein had established himself as a famous scientist, he replied to a friend's request for a description of his thought processes:

> The words of the language, as they are written or spoken, do not seem to play any role in my mechanisms of thought. The psychological entities which seem to serve as elements in thought are certain signs or more or less clear images which can be voluntarily reproduced and combined. There is, of course, a certain connection between these elements and relevant logical concepts. It is also clear that the desire to arrive finally at logically connected concepts is the emotional basis of this rather vague play with the above mentioned elements. But taken from a psychological viewpoint, this combinatory play seems to be the essential feature in productive thought — before there is any connection with logical construction in words or other kinds of signs which can be communicated to others.

The above mentioned elements are in my case, visual and some of muscular type. Conventional words or other signs have to be sought for laboriously only in a secondary stage, when the mentioned associative play is sufficiently established and can be reproduced at will.[23]

A person whose thought processes were of this sort might not function particularly well in a school where concepts are dealt with predominantly through the medium of the spoken and written word.

Another source of Einstein's difficulties was his poor memory for details. A friend of his parents once told them their son "will never amount to anything because he can't remember anything." His tendency to forget his key would result in waking up his landlady late at night, calling out, "It's Einstein — I've forgotten my key again."[24] To the extent that school requires memory for details, how could he avoid being in trouble with teachers?

Einstein was a nonconformist who had a special appreciation for intuitive, imaginative thinking. The only school teacher he could remember appreciating had a way of getting students to think for themselves. This was in contrast to other teachers whom he saw as expecting military obedience.[25] We get a picture of a young man possessing unusual spatial-thought processes, somewhat slow in verbal and memory skills, and with a tendency to have strong emotional reactions that could get him into trouble with teachers. Memories of his experience would lead Einstein to say in later life that "the teachers in the elementary school appeared to me like sargeants and in the gymnasium the teachers were like lieutenants."[26]

Einstein managed to reenter the academic world through the Swiss Federal Polytechnic School, but he never did adapt to this world. He was considered undisciplined in his studies and often lost track of technical details in his work. One professor tried to prevent him from studying theoretical physics. When Einstein finished the course work, none of the professors would take him as an assistant. This prevented him from following the usual route to an academic career. Through this period of his life, he felt that he had been "abandoned by everyone, standing at a loss on the threshold of life."[27] For the next two years, four different temporary jobs provided him a living while he wrote letters to physics professors all over Europe requesting an assistant's position. None would have him. Finally, he landed a regular job as a clerk in the Swiss patent office. It wasn't until a few years later, when his paper on the special theory of relativity was published, that Einstein succeeded in convincing anyone in the academic world that he had something of value to offer.

VIRGINIA WOOLF

It is speculative to consider the possibility that people who did not make a name for themselves in graphic, spatially dominated professions might nevertheless have been spatial children. The direct evidence of accomplishment in spatial skills is not present, and one must work from less direct evidence. It would not be appropriate, however, to suggest that spatial children can only achieve in spatially dominated professions or that spatial skills are of no value outside those professions. Spatial ability relates to the broader capacity for seeing patterns and connections. This can be of value in any profession.

The information from the childhood of Virginia Woolf is certainly not as convincing as that from the childhoods of Einstein and Picasso, but the possibilities it suggests make the case equally interesting. Virginia Woolf, born in 1882, grew up in a comfortable, upper middle-class English family noted for some literary accomplishment. Her father, Leslie Stephen, was a prolific writer and an editor of a literary magazine. The surroundings were ideal for the development of the verbally precocious child, which Woolf eventually became. But this was not her initial approach to life. Her early verbal development was unusually slow. Her sister Vanessa wrote a memorial recalling events of their childhood together: "She cannot have been more than two, and I therefore only about four and a half. But it is a vivid memory to me. How worried I was too, not much later, because she couldn't speak clearly; I feared she would never do so, which would certainly have been a misfortune."[28]

In a biographical account, Woolf's nephew, Quentin Bell, reports that this was of considerable concern to her parents.[29] Woolf's older half sister, Laura, suffered a lifelong schizophrenia that had aspects of communication difficulties. For the parents to fear that Virginia was headed in that direction was natural.

This course of development changed abruptly when Woolf was three, and from that point on there is no evidence of any inordinate difficulties with language. However, an academic evaluation of her abilities was never part of her experience. Woolf (1976)* stated, "Owing partly to the fact that I was never at school, never competed in any way with children of my own age, I have never been able to compare my gifts and defects with other people's."[30] It was still the custom in the late 1800s for girls to receive their schooling at home, and the education of the Stephen girls was quite informal. Woolf was noted for enjoying reading and writing, but no record of what this actually entailed seems to be available. Considering the difficulties that were involved in editing her adult literary works for errors in writing mechanics, it is entirely possible that her childhood writing might have been more noted for the enjoyment it gave a girl who was expected to have no particular scholarly ambitions than for its technical adequacy.

More interesting are the conjectures about her thought processes. There is evidence that sensory images may have been so dominant and refined in her early experience that she had difficulty connecting those images to words and finding the correct words to relate the impressions. Years later she could recall the impressions accordingly. "The strength of these pictures — but sight was always then so much mixed with sound that picture is not the right word — the strength anyhow of these impressions makes me again digress. Those moments — in the nursery, on the road to the beach — can still be more real than the present moment."[31] There were times in her youth when she found it difficult using words to represent sense impressions.[32] The imagery would take control, and her mind would involuntarily create perceptions without verbal associations. This imagery became the creative basis for her later work, what she called *scene making*. She stated, "Whatever the reason may be, I find that scene making is my natural way of marking the past. Always a scene has arranged itself; representative: enduring. . . . Is this liability to scenes the origin of my writing impulse? . . . Obviously I have developed the faculty, because, in all the writing I have done, I have almost always had to make a scene, even when I am writing about a person; I must find a representative scene in their lives."[33]

Although this became the basis for her creative work, there were also times when she felt that words and language were not a sufficient means to convey the meanings she felt. Language became

---

*From Virginia Woolf, *Moments of Being,* 1976. Courtesy of the Hogarth Press, London, England, and Harcourt Brace Jovanovich, Inc., New York.

superficial and disconnected from the imagery of her mind.[34] The scenes that seemed to break automatically in upon her mind became the most real, the most permanent aspect of her being. She reported, "This confirms me in my instinctive notion: (it will not bear arguing about; it is irrational) the sensation that we are sealed vessels afloat on what it is convenient to call reality; and at some moments, the sealing matter cracks; in floods reality; that is, these scenes — for why do they survive undamaged year after year unless they are made of something comparatively permanent?"[35]

As for formal language, for a person who wrote so much, and who became so distinguished for her literary work, she was perhaps unusual in never having the inclination, patience, and perhaps knowledge to perfect her own work. One editor, after laboring long over one of her posthumously published works, complained somewhat of the effort and of the unease at being forced to take considerable liberties in order to make the work of a genius seem intelligible:

> In early drafts, Virginia Woolf's practice regarding punctuation, spelling and capitalization was highly erratic and she often used abbreviations which never appeared in her published work. On occasion, obvious oversights coupled with typing mistakes and incomplete or hastily made corrections have resulted in a profusion of errors; at others, the careful attention to these matters which characterizes her published works is evident. It was Virginia Woolf's practice to submit her work to her husband, Leonard, for revision of these details and he, in publishing her posthumous works, did not hesitate, as he writes in the editorial preface to *The Death of the Moth* "to punctuate" the essays and correct obvious verbal mistakes.[36]

We might say that Virginia Woolf was never quite at home in the world of formal language, and that scene making was her most natural mode of cognition.

AUGUSTE RODIN

Rodin was born in 1840 in the village of Mouffetard on the outskirts of Paris. His father had a strong religious and moral bent, so much so that he spent several years with the Brotherhood of the Christian Doctrine before settling on a career as a minor police official. Rodin's mother was equally devout. Neither parent had any sympathy for the idea of Rodin becoming an artist; a career they felt was inevitably associated with Bohemianism. The financial instability of the artist's life had nothing that a cautious, upright middle-class family could relate to.

But artistry was key to the personality of young Rodin. As the adult Rodin recalled it, he drew from as early an age as he could remember. The local grocer would wrap prunes in the pages of old magazines, and Rodin would retrieve the pages, using the illustrations as his first models.[37] Much of his time in school was spent drawing. This contributed to an elementary school experience that could be characterized as a total failure.

Rodin first attended the Ecoles Chretiennes, a religious school noted for its progressive methods of teaching young children. Whatever the reputation of the school, it could do nothing for Rodin. His capacity for reading and writing was virtually not present. When Rodin reached age nine, the family, in desperation, made other arrangements. An uncle ran a small boarding school in Beauvais. The school had the discipline of a military academy. That discipline, combined with the special attention to be given by the uncle would surely get Rodin in line and shape up his academic skills. But it was not to be. Four years at the boarding school left Rodin as backward as before. "He seemed to be genuinely retarded. His dictation was riddled with crass spelling-mistakes. He never succeeded in learning Latin like the others, and his mathematics were nonexistent."[38] Rodin returned home as much a failure as before. For his father, who had built his own security on petty academic knowledge, this meant disaster. What would Rodin do for a living?

The personality of young Rodin may have ill-suited him for the austere boarding school as much as his intellectual backwardness. The boys in the school, suffering the conditions of the harsh discipline, were as brutish to each other as they were miserable. This affected the sensitive, retiring Rodin to the extent that he was seen as a quiet loner having little to do with the rough and tumble affairs of the other boys. "He loitered in the corner of the play-ground, a silent and solitary figure, and dreaded the dormitory's lack of privacy."[39]

Whatever his lack of assertiveness in social situations, he was quite determined in one thing: the desire to be an artist. When Rodin returned home with the disgrace of his academic failure, the natural topic of discussion surrounding the thirteen-year-old boy was the method by which he would come to support himself. Rodin was determined to study art. His father had no good ideas for what else Rodin might do, but artistry was certainly not considered a reasonable way to make a living. The difference of opinion became the point of heated family discussions.

Fortunately for Rodin's case, there was a streak of romanticism in the family along with the middle-class virtues. His mother was a dour woman, but her own family had a bent for art, and two of her nephews were studying art with their parents' support. Rodin's sister, Maria, came down firmly on his side, arguing that if art was the only thing he enjoyed, he should just as well be allowed a chance to make a career of it. The father gave in, perhaps thinking that after Rodin had come to realize for himself the impracticality of art, he would agree to a more useful vocation.

Rodin spent three years studying at the Ecole gratuite de dessin in Paris, which was popularly called the Petite Ecole to distinguish it from the more prestigious Grande Ecole des Beaux-Arts. He became a dedicated student, spending virtually all of his time developing his craft — mornings at the school, afternoons at galleries and libraries, and evenings in more classes.[40] The school prepared him to be a craftsman who might make a living at practical applications of the arts. But when his studies at the Petite Ecole were complete, he had ambitions to go on to more refined studies at the Grande Ecole. His parents, after already supporting him in art studies for three years, balked, wondering again where it would all lead. Again, sister Maria backed her brother, insisting that after he had worked so hard at developing his skills, he shouldn't be denied the chance to continue.

However, admission to the Grande Ecole involved much more than convincing his parents. It was the most competitive school in France, and many fine artists were never admitted. The family decided that an authority in sculpture should be consulted to see what Rodin's real prospects might be. Rodin pulled a cartload of his work to the door of Maindron, the most successful sculptor in Paris, for a quick assessment. Maindron was either impressed or sympathetic to the young man's dreams. Rodin was encouraged to study at the Grande Ecole.

Receiving the backing of the old sculptor was almost certainly a fortunate break in the development of the career of Auguste Rodin, because it encouraged him to continue with his dreams in spite of never being admitted to the Grande Ecole. Rodin applied once to the Grande Ecole and was rejected. He applied a second time, and was rejected. His determination led to a third application, and again, he was denied admission. Finally, in frustration he gave up. Auguste Rodin would later come to realize that being rejected by the Grande Ecole was not as important as he once thought and that his rejection was perhaps due to an inherent gulf between his natural artistic style and the pedantic style of the establishment art world. But this must have been a stressful time for the young, ambitious art student. Only his own determination and many years of struggle among the lower ranks of artists would see him through to finding the most successful career in the history of sculpture.

REFERENCES

1. Much of the information on Reuben was graciously provided by his parents.
2. Fadely, J.L., and Hosler, V.N. *Understanding the Alpha Child at Home and School.* Springfield, Ill.: Charles C Thomas, Publisher, 1979, p. 177.
3. Nilda was gracious in being interviewed concerning this observation on her development.
4. The information on Mary Laycock was graciously provided in a special communication from Mary.
5. Laycock, M., and Watson, G. *The Fabric of Mathematics.* Hayward, Calif.: Activities Resources Company, 1975.
6. O'Brian, P. *Picasso.* New York: G.P. Putnam's Sons, 1976, p. 23.
7. *Ibid.,* p. 25.
8. *Ibid.,* p. 25.
9. Bannatyne, A. *Language, Reading and Learning Disabilities.* Springfield, Ill.: Charles C Thomas, Publisher, 1971, p. 646.
10. O'Brian, *op. cit.,* p. 35.
11. O'Brian, *op. cit.,* p. 26.
12. O'Brian, *op. cit.,* p. 38.
13. Clark, R.W. *Einstein.* New York: Avon Books, 1971, pp. 29-30.
14. *Ibid.,* p. 30.
15. Talmey, M. *The Relativity Theory Simplified and the Formative Period of its Inventor.* New York: 1932.
16. *Ibid.,* p. 164.
17. Letter from Albert Einstein to Casar Koch. Translated by Jagdish Mehra.
18. Clark, *op. cit.,* p. 42.
19. Clark, *op. cit.,* p. 27.
20. Clark, *op. cit.,* p. 39.
21. Clark, *op. cit.,* p. 27.
22. Clark, *op. cit.,* p. 73.

23. Letter from Albert Einstein to Jacques Hadamard. Reproduced in Ghiselin, B. *The Creative Process.* New York: Mentor Books, 1952, p. 43.
24. Clark, *op. cit.,* p. 50.
25. Clark, *op. cit.,* p. 33.
26. Clark, *op. cit.,* p. 31.
27. Clark, *op. cit.,* p. 62.
28. Bell, V. *Notes on Virginia's Childhood.* New York: A Memorial Statement, 1974, unpaged.
29. Bell, Q. *Virginia Woolf.* New York: Harcourt Brace Jovanovich, 1972, p. 22.
30. Woolf, V. *Moments of Being.* Sussex, England: Sussex University Press, 1976, p. 65.
31. *Ibid.,* p. 67.
32. Love, J.L. *Virginia Woolf: Sources of Madness and Art.* Berkeley, Calif.: University of California Press, 1977, p. 217.
33. Woolf, *op. cit.,* p. 122.
34. Love, *op. cit.,* p. 272.
35. Woolf, *op. cit.,* p. 122.
36. Schulkind, J. Editor's note. In Woolf, V. *Moments of Being.* Sussex, England: Sussex University Press, 1976, p. 9.
37. Champigneulle, B. *Rodin.* New York: Oxford University Press, 1980, p. 12.
38. *Ibid.,* p. 12.
39. *Ibid.,* p. 12.
40. *Ibid.,* pp. 14-15.

Chapter 5

TWO HEMISPHERES

OUR DIVIDED EXISTENCE

GRASP of the nature of our existence is to some extent separated into the recognition of two types of phenomena. One of these involves objects, and the other involves action. The two most basic parts of speech, nouns (dogs) and verbs (run), help us represent and interconnect the two. Objects have parts and consistent ways in which the parts are connected. Recognition of consistent patterns in the parts and connections allows one type of object to be distinguished from another. The pattern allows objects to be represented in a rather complete, static form as a drawing or a sculpture. This kind of representation is complete in an holistic way, out can only catch objects at one moment in the active flow of reality. In that sense, static representation is limited. It does not deal with action.

Action can also be represented. But since action consists of a flow of a succession of moments in the life of objects, it cannot be so easily depicted in a complete manner. A music score, for example, could be thought of as a representation of a sequence of action. However, it is very incomplete. It is just marks on a piece of paper. It does not begin to completely show a musician or set of musicians each of the infinitely many successions of positions that make up the playing of a song. If musicians did not possess a complex set of understandings about the behavior they must undertake to produce the series of sounds implied by the score, a set of understandings that go far beyond what any nonmusician could make out from the bare notes on a sheet of paper, music notation could hardly lead to the producton of a recognizable song. A flow of action is so complex that recording it requires some special recording system, such as writing or music notation in which a whole host of assumed meanings can be presented in a simple, symbolic, sequential form. The notation systems that have evolved for recording dance movements demon-

102

strate how difficult it is to record action when one needs to approach recording the full details of the action. Most dancers concur that a completely satisfactory notation system has not yet been developed.

It would not be correct to imply that these two ways of looking at phenomena — the holistic-graphic representation of objects and the sequential-detailed representation of action — are completely separate. They are actually very much intertwined. For example, when a scientist draws the orbit of a planet around the sun, each infinitely small point in the drawing represents a distinct moment in the action sequence of the planet. The drawing of the orbit allows the total collection of these moments to be dealt with almost as if, collectively speaking, they were a whole object like a ring. Some of the greatest achievements of man have derived from the capacity to grasp the pattern in a representative sequence of action and then to find a way to graphically depict the pattern of action as if it were a whole. Much of the field of mathematics involves the search for ways in which the underlying patterns in sets of details can be represented in a generalizable, often graphic, form.

Sometimes sequences of behavior are dealt with as if they constituted a whole that can hardly be separated. A basketball player doing a lay-up is performing a sequence of behaviors that is so welded together by repeated practice that each action can hardly be separated out from the whole pattern. When we sing a well-known song, each note, each word, is so tied together that the omission of any note or word immediately signals that something is missing. One becomes aware of how difficult it is to deliberately omit parts of a song when signing the children's song *There Was a Dog Named Bingo*, in which the omission of parts of the song is turned into a game requiring careful concentration.

Just as whole patterns come to convey the essence of some sequence of action, sequences of detailed action can be used to represent the qualities of a whole thing. A picture in a newspaper consists of rows of small light or dark dots, which, when put together, create the pictures of objects. These pictures are sent around the world through transmission of the sequence of dots. The same principle is used in the transmission of television signals in which the sequential transmission of rows of dots is done so quickly that the motion of objects can be recreated.

In spite of the interconnected nature of holistic-graphic representation and sequential-detailed representation, they evidently are so distinct that they require two different ways of being processed by the nerve cells in our brains. This is a conclusion that brain researchers arrived at after more than a century of observing the behavioral manifestations of the two distinct kinds of thinking. Although not enough is known about the ways this research relates to the way children think and learn, it is clear that the connections are beginning to be made; it is important for all educators to have a knowledge of this research.

THE HISTORICAL DEVELOPMENT
OF CEREBRAL ASYMMETRY RESEARCH

The upper and outermost surface parts of our brains, those parts covered by winding, wavy convolutions, are responsible for many of our most intellectual processes. These outer parts are called the *cerebral cortex*. There are several rather deep, separating grooves running through the cortex that divide it into sections that can be readily recognized by neurosurgeons and others who have the opportunity to get inside our skulls. The principal separating groove runs through the middle of the cortex from the forehead to the back of our heads. It makes the most distinct division of the cortex such that the two resulting sides have come to be called the left and right hemispheres.

It wasn't until the 1860s and 1870s that this division began to take on psychological significance. Paul Broca, a French neurosurgeon, discovered that when the left hemisphere suffered injury or disease in the front, temple area, a person would have problems with speaking. Speech would be slow and labored. It might take on a simplified form in which words would be left out of sentences or the endings of words would be dropped from speech. A patient might get confused trying to repeat a special phrase like, "No doubt about it." This difficulty is sometimes called *expressive aphasia,* and in honor of the discovery of its relationship to brain injury, the specified part of our brains is now called *Broca's Area.* Broca also discovered that a similar injury to the right side of the brain tended to not result in this speech difficulty.

About ten years after Broca's discovery, a brilliant young German neurologist, Carl Wernicke, found that a different kind of aphasia was caused by injury to another left hemisphere area behind the ear. This aphasia is characterized by associational problems. The connection between words and their meaning is lost. The person may be fluent in speech, but often can't find the names of objects he is attempting to talk about. Empty words or phrases such as *thing* or *what's-his-face* are used, or objects might be described, e.g. "the thing you eat with." For his discovery of this form of aphasia, this part of the left hemisphere is called *Wernicke's Area*. Again, it was demonstrated that an injury to the same location on the right hemisphere tended to not result in the associational aphasia.

In the century since the discoveries of Broca and Wernicke, neurologists have achieved considerable sophistication in understanding the specialization of cortex areas for language use — also for the way these areas hang together. Most of this knowledge focuses on the left hemisphere. Because intellectual work relies heavily on the use of language, those who studied brain functioning came to think of the left hemisphere as being responsible for intellectual processes, and hence the "dominant" or "major" hemisphere. Since little was known about the functioning of the right hemisphere, it was called the "minor" hemisphere. This has remained the accepted terminology up to the present time.

In spite of the fact that most interest was focused on the language dominant left hemisphere, almost from the time of Broca and Wernicke, there have been a few scientists who took special interest in the psychological consequences of disease to the right hemisphere. In the 1870s, the British neurosurgeon Hughlings Jackson described a patient with a tumor in the back part of the right hemisphere. The woman suffered from directional disorientation, difficulty in recognizing persons and places, and debilitation in dressing herself. Jackson evidently was one who placed great store on the intellectual value of being in touch with the physical world around oneself as opposed to being able to use words. He went so far as to suggest that the skills of the right hemisphere are intellectually more significant than those of the verbal left. He said, "The posterior lobes are the seat of the most intellectual processes. This is in effect saying that they are the seat of visual ideation, for most of our mental operations are carried on in visual ideas. I think too that the right posterior lobe is the leading side."[1] Jackson's preference for the right hemisphere is interesting. It is perhaps an indication that he was a visual-spatial thinker. Many good surgeons are.

Although there were many scattered reports during the latter part of the nineteenth century and the early part of the twentieth century of people who suffered loss of directional orientation, confusion in locating objects in space, and a general loss of geographic sense as a result of right hemisphere disease or injury, Jackson's suggestion of the importance of the right hemisphere in intellectual processes was generally not taken with any seriousness.[2] During the 1930s and 1940s, interest in the special abilities of the right hemisphere began to grow.[3] In 1935, Weisenburg and McBride reported on a study in which patients with right hemisphere lesions were compared to those with left hemisphere lesions. Those with right hemisphere lesions were significantly impaired in many nonverbal tasks even though their verbal abilities were nearly normal. In 1936, Hebb described a patient in whom a portion of the right hemisphere was removed. The patient was superior in verbal intelligence but very defective in visual form perception, in spatial construction tests, and in haptic recognition (recognition of objects when they can only be handled but not seen). And in 1941, a British neurosurgeon by the unlikely name of Brain published an extensive description of the difficulties of patients with disease or injury of the right hemisphere. Some patients were so spatially disoriented they would get lost in their own homes. They might correctly describe in verbal terms the relationship between places and objects. At the same time, they were unable to act with appropriate orientation in relation to those places and objects. One patient would get lost going from his bedroom to his sitting room. He would become upset by the mistake. He could describe perfectly the steps for going from one room to the other. He just couldn't follow his own directions. Some of Brain's patients were unable to dress themselves. They might put their clothes on backward or upside down. Elaborate strategies would be created to help them get dressed. Even with considerable training, a task that would seem easy to most people was difficult and tedious.

These reports by Weisenburg, McBride, Hebb, and Brain probably should have been the focus of greater interest, and they should have motivated more studies on the localization of human abilities within the brain. However, this research was going on before psychologists like Piaget had established the importance of spatial knowledge in intellectual processes and at a time when many scholars thought that verbal reasoning was the primary medium of all intellectual thought.[4]

SPERRY'S SPLIT-BRAIN PATIENTS

The biggest boost to research on hemispheric asymmetry came in the early 1950s when Ronald Myers and Roger Sperry carried out a fascinating line of research involving a cat. (Perhaps the cat didn't think it was so fascinating.) Myers and Sperry cut the main nerve connections between the left and right hemispheres of the cat's brain. This large bundle of connections is called the *corpus callosum*. In this surgery, they also divided the optic chiasm so that images entering the left eye would only go to the left hemisphere and images entering the right eye would only go to the right hemisphere.

The cat's behavior was not seriously affected by the surgery. A learning experiment, however, revealed to Myers and Sperry that after the corpus callosum surgery, the cat essentially had two separately functioning brains. In this experiment, one of the cat's eyes was covered with a patch, and the cat was taught to carry out a task through rewarded conditioning, i.e. a little bit of cat food after each correct performance. When the eye patch was shifted to the other eye, so that all visual information was now going to the other side of the brain, the cat showed no evidence of ever having learned the task. This indicated that the corpus callosum was the principal means by which information was passed from one hemisphere to the other. It also indicated that the two hemispheres could operate quite independently of each other, and that loss of the corpus callosum connections was not life-threatening to the animal.[5]

This discovery led to another creative idea. It was known that serious epileptic seizures involve an uncontrolled firing of nerve cells back and forth between the two hemispheres. Since animals could live without the corpus callosum connections, it was thought that in cases where a person's life was unbearably debilitated by seizures, cutting the connections might limit the uncontrolled firing. The hunch was correct. When surgeons began to carry out this procedure, they found that it led to the near complete elimination of all seizures. While Doctors Vogel and Bogen at the California College of Medicine were performing the surgery, Sperry and Michael Gazzaniga at the California Institute of Technology had the opportunity to study how it affected the behavior of the patients.

Just as the lack of corpus callosum connections appeared not to affect the life adjustment of Sperry's cat, observation of the patients indicated they were also affected little by the loss of the connections. They acted much the same and had very much the same competencies as before the surgery. After more careful observation, however, it became clear that the patients had no verbal recognition of events involving the left side of their bodies. When a patient brushed against something with the left side of his body, there was no verbal report that it happened. When an object was placed in the left hand, the patient would deny that it was there. The left side of the body, which is largely controlled by the nonverbal right hemisphere, was receiving no recognition by the verbal left hemisphere of its existence. When a light was flashed in the left visual field of the patient, he didn't report that it had happened. However, when the patient was allowed to point to the place in the left field where the light had flashed, he could do so. Clearly, the right hemisphere knew what was happening, but it had no means for talking about what it knew.[6]

These observations led Sperry and Gazzaniga to carry out a series of investigations of "split-brain" behavior. In some cases, they would have patients put their hands under a screen; then the researchers would place an object in either the left hand or the right hand. When a patient explored an object with his right hand (largely controlled by the left hemisphere), he could name it. When he held the object in the left hand (right hemisphere), he couldn't name the object, but he could point to a picture of it. If the patient was shown a picture of an object with his left hand, he could pick it out from a group of other objects. The right hemisphere might even make associations. If shown the picture of a cigarette, it will guide the left hand in picking out an ash tray from among nonassociated objects.

Sperry and Gazzaniga found some facility for written language in the right hemisphere. They would use a device called a tachistoscope, which makes a precisely timed flash of a picture or word on a projection screen. If a split-brain patient is looking straightforward and information is flashed on the left side of the screen, it will go only to the right hemisphere, and vice versa. For some patients, if a word like *pencil* was flashed to the right hemisphere, they would be able to find a pencil from among other objects even when they couldn't name the pencil. However, this verbal knowledge was very limited in the right hemisphere. If a verb like *smile* or *frown* were flashed to the right hemisphere, the patients would be unable to carry out the instruction or to pick out a picture of someone smiling or frowning.[7]

There were some tasks that the right hemisphere (left hand) could carry out with much greater facility than the left. When the split-brain patients were given an activity in which a set of blocks were to be arranged according to a design in a picture, the left hand carried out the task with ease, while the right hand could not do it. The same difference occurred in design copying.

DIFFERENCES IN SIGHT, SOUND, AND TACTILE PERCEPTION

This line of research by Myers, Sperry, Gazzaniga, Bogen, and Vogel was such a dramatic demonstration of separate capacities in the two hemispheres of the human brain that innumerable research studies on hemispheric asymmetry have followed, and the popular literature on its meaning has abounded. Most studies have involved people with an intact corpus callosum. Under this usual condition, study of hemispheric asymmetry is more difficult to carry out because communication across the corpus callosum is so fast that each hemisphere is almost instantaneously privy to information given to the other. Nevertheless, differences have been found.

Some studies have focused on visual differences. Durnford has carried out experiments in which people are asked to match sloping lines flashed on a tachistoscope to those on a sheet of paper. Those flashed in the left visual field (right hemisphere) are more accurately matched than those flashed in the right visual field.[8] Durnford also found the distance judgments of the right hemisphere to be more accurate.

Differences between the hemispheres have been found in the perception of sound. A technique called dichotic listening allows for two different sounds to be delivered to the two ears at the same time. The connections from the ears to the two hemispheres are not quite the same as those from the eyes. A sound coming into the left ear will be received more distinctly by the right hemisphere than the left, but the crossed nature of the connections are not as distinct as those in vision. To some extent, a person will hear the same sounds in the two hemispheres. Nevertheless, distinctions can be detected in the kinds of sounds each hemisphere is most capable of interpreting. Kimura simultaneously presented two different digit names (3 and 8) to the two ears. Those presented to the right ear tended to be reported as heard more than those presented to the left ear. The left hemisphere was evidently more sensitive in the reception of verbal information.[9] In a subsequent piece of research, Knox and Kimura found that when roughly comparable non-verbal sounds (car starting or water pouring) were presented, those going to the left ear were more often reported as heard. The right hemisphere would appear to be more sensitive in interpreting natural sounds.[10]

Another way we have of interpreting the events in the world around us is through touching and feeling, i.e. tactile or haptic perception. It has long been known that the right hemisphere has a special strength in tactile perception. In the early part of this century, those who worked at teaching blind children to read through the Braille system discovered that the children were often able to read more accurately with the left hand than with the right.[11] This seemed surprising to neurologists. Since tactile perception is rather clearly crossed from hand to cerebral hemisphere (the right hemisphere receiving information from the left hand), and since the left hemisphere is the more verbal hemisphere, it seemed more logical that the right hand would be the Braille reading hand. The observations, however, went quite consistently in the other direction. In 1971, Hermelin and O'Connor reported on an experiment in which the left hand speed-reading scores of blind children were significantly faster than their right hand scores.[12] They found one child who had injured his left hand, which he called his reading hand, and was unable to read. Evidently, the pattern recognition aspects of Braille reading are crucial for initial perception. Whether the initial tactile perceptions are then immediately transferred from the right hemisphere to the left for linguistic interpretation is not known. Considering the ability of the left hemisphere for interpreting grammatical constructions, one might assume that something like this occurs. Tactile perception of patterns, even linguistically meaningful ones, is clearly quite dependent on the pattern recognition abilities of the right hemisphere.

In research involving sighted children, Kimura has found right hemisphere superiority for visual perception of dot patterns similar to those used in Braille reading.[13] Kimura would tachistoscopically flash these dot patterns to either the left or right visual field, and then would test for the accuracy of perception. Witelson has shown that if sighted, but blindfolded, children explore nonsense shapes with their hands and then are asked to identify the shapes in a visual display, those shapes explored with the left hand will be more accurately identified.[14] Ingram has shown that children are more accurate in copying demonstrated hand positions with their left hand than with their right; this included lifting designated fingers, bending joints, and creating spaces between fingers.[15] There is no doubt that the right hemisphere is more accurate than the left in the tactile perception of patterns, and in the correct perception of body positioning.

BEYOND LANGUAGE VS. GRAPHICS

This line of research involving language use and involving sight, sound, and tactile perception begins to give a clear picture of the separate natures of the two hemispheres. The left hemisphere is specialized for language, for comprehension and production of speech; and especially for subtle conventions in the grammatical sequencing of language. The right hemisphere, on the other hand, has a specialization for recognition and understanding of graphic designs and spatial relationships and for recognizing patterns of sounds that have naturalistic meaning. The right hemisphere can become helpful in language processes when these processes involve recognition of spatial patterns, such as Braille dot patterns. The language comprehension ability of the right hemisphere is mostly limited to nouns, the part of speech that refers to the kinds of graphic objects that the right hemisphere is most adept at understanding. The right hemisphere has little facility for understanding other parts of speech that enter into the complete sequencing conventions of language, e.g. verbs, adjectives, and adverbs.

We need to proceed with caution, however, lest we make the mistake of concluding that the only distinction in the hemispheres is a specialization for language in one and graphic understanding in the other. We need to look further at the research, and particularly at distinctions in kinds of language, areas of musical skill, and areas of graphic ability.

In the language area, although the right hemisphere is inefficient at most language skills, it is quite capable in others. For example, after a person's usual capacity to carry on a conversation has been interrupted by left hemisphere disease or injury, very often the person retains an established knowledge of poetry or other emotionally meaningful sequences of language, sequences that hang together in holistic ways.[16] In such cases, the person also retains a capacity to use descriptive words and phrases to communicate desires or thoughts. This would indicate that the right hemisphere processes language related to the qualities of objects. Head put it this way: "When an aphasic (one who has difficulty speaking) cannot employ more abstract terms, he often uses descriptive phrases, similes, and metaphorical expressions in an appropriate manner."[17] This simple, descriptive approach to language is distinguished from what Bogen calls propositional speech that is debilitated by the left hemisphere injury, i.e. "words referring to one another in a particular manner so that each modifies the meaning of the other."[18] The person loses the ability to quickly construct lengthy, subtle sequences of words that are considered appropriate to each given circumstance.

There seems to be a similar distinction in the skills related to music. As long ago as 1745, Dalin described a patient who had had a stroke in the left hemisphere and retained an ability to sing and use other expressive modes.

> He had an attack of a violent illness which resulted in a paralysis of the entire right side of the body and complete loss of speech. . . . He can sing certain hymns, which he had learned before he became ill, as clearly and distinctly as any healthy person. However, it should be noted that at the beginning of the hymn he has to be helped a little by some other person singing with him. Similarly, with the same type of help, he can recite certain prayers without singing, but with a certain rhythm and in a high pitched, shouting tone. Yet, this man is dumb, cannot say a single word except "yes" and has to communicate by making signs with his hand.[19]

Left hemisphere brain damage does debilitate the use of the more formal, intellectual musical skills, such as reading and writing music. In 1926, Head described patients with left hemisphere injury who had no difficulty with "melody and the recognition of time and tune," but did have difficulty in "reading the notes of the music."[20] In 1962, Hecaen compared music abilities of people who had either left or right hemisphere lesions. Those with left hemisphere lesions suffered from a "disorganization of musical understanding," while those with right hemisphere lesions suffered from a difficulty in the "recognition of musical sounds."[21] Milner gave the Seashore Music Tests to people who had part of either their left or right hemispheres surgically removed. She found that the memory of people for tones was seriously affected by removal of right hemisphere tissue, but not particularly affected by removal of left hemisphere tissue.[22] Kimura and Shankweiler have both found evidence for superior melody recognition in the right hemisphere.[23]

Alajouanine has described the way a stroke affected the famous composer Ravel. He was virtually incapacitated in recognizing musical notation and in playing the piano if he needed to sight read a score. On the other hand, his sense of melody, rhythm, and style were unaffected, and he could play the piano or sing from memory. Although Ravel's productive career was ended by his inability to communicate to others through music notation, "his artistic sensibility does not seem to be in the least altered."[24] There are reports of others with a similar malady who have carried on in spite of the difficulty. Luria described the case of a composer who wrote some of his best works after a left hemisphere stroke caused limitations in the use of language. Critchley described a patient suffering from a similar difficulty who continued to conduct his own orchestra.[25]

The distinction we seem to be faced with in music is similar to that in language. The more formal, detailed aspects of music that place music within conventions, which can be precisely communicated from one person to another, are dependent on the left hemisphere. Those aspects that derive their meaningfulness from the sense that each note fits a simultaneously felt larger context of the tune or song are dependent on the right hemisphere. Pitch, rhythm, and tone are meaningful within the larger context. One note by itself has little meaning. Its meaning derives from its relation to others in a tune. An *A* note officially consists of a 440 cycle per second vibration. But this knowledge is not what makes it meaningful in music. An *A* has a certain felt relationship to a *B* note, and it is the whole system of patterning in the relationships between notes that gives each its significance. Play one sour note and it may ruin the song, not because there is anything inherently wrong with the note itself (it might be a perfectly nice note) but because it doesn't fit into the pattern of relationships between notes in the tune as holistically felt.

In this sense, music is similar to spatial understanding. Every detail has certain relationships to every other detail, and the simultaneous grasp of this at any moment is what gives beauty to the whole. Howard Gardner pointed out that Mozart explained his thought processes in this way. The holistic patterns that he could see in his mind's eye were inspirational beyond explanation. "All this fires my soul, and provided I am not disturbed, my subject enlarges itself, becomes methodized and defined, and the whole, though it be long, stands almost complete and finished in my mind, so that I can survey it like a fine picture or a beautiful statue, at a glance. Nor do I hear in my imagination the parts successively, but I hear them, as it were, all at once. What a delight this is I cannot tell."[26] Perhaps some of Mozart's creative powers derived from his sensitivity to the structured, patterned aspects of music — the relationships that hold a piece of music together.

Just as distinctions can be made between two different approaches in both language and music, a similar distinction can be made in graphics. When Gazzaniga and Bogen asked split-brain patients to reproduce block arrangements with their left hand (controlled by their right hemisphere), the patients were able to do this much better than with their right hand. However, it isn't that the left hemisphere has no figural or graphic knowledge. When the patients were asked to copy simple drawings, the copies attempted by the right hand were rather precise in details. The problem was that the pictures produced by the right hand didn't come very close to the overall structure of the original.[27] The copies produced by the left hand came much closer to matching the overall structure, but they were rather imprecise in detail (Figure 5-1).

Even though the left hemisphere does have abilities that are important for achieving detailed precision in graphic design, it is appropriate to consider the right hemisphere to be the spatially competent hemisphere because sensitivity to the overall gestalt is the essence of spatial awareness. In Smith's factor analytic studies of spatial ability, the one common element in all spatial tasks was this grasp of the total configuration of relationships by which objects hang together and relate to each other. In Smith's words, "Success in the item must depend critically on an ability to retain and recognize (or reproduce) a configuration as an organized whole. . . . Success or failure in an item also depends critically on gestalt — or form —

EXAMPLE   LEFT HAND   RIGHT HAND

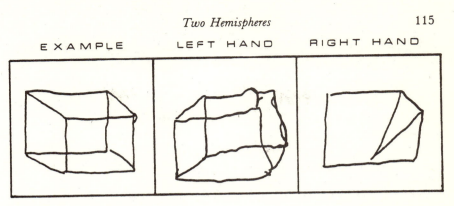

Figure 5-1. The drawings of one of Michael S. Gazzaniga's split-brain patients in reproducing the example pattern with the left hand and the right hand. From Michael S. Gazzaniga, The split brain in man, *Scientific American 217*, 2:28, August 1967. Courtesy of Gazzaniga.

perception. . . . It is only when the complexity is of a kind which compels the subject to rely on the perception of a configuration as a whole that the test involves K."[28]

For Piaget, this grasp of the gestalt was the end result of the development of formal operational thinking within the spatial realm. This was true whether the operations were based on projective understanding or on Euclidean understanding.

GRASP OF THE GESTALT IN DIVERSE SYSTEMS

A consistent conclusion is derived from the cerebral asymmetry research. Whether we are dealing with the distinction between propositional language (left hemisphere), vs. poetic, metaphoric language (right hemisphere), the distinction between the conventions of musical notation (left hemisphere) vs. the sense of tonal and rhythmic structure (right hemisphere), or the distinction between the grasp of detail in graphic design (left hemisphere) vs. the sense of overall structure in graphic design (right hemisphere), the differences are similar. The left hemisphere is good at dealing with the precise details that are so important in conventional ways of approaching the world. Whether we are spelling a word, reading a note on a music score, or constructing an angle, we are concerned with the cultural conventions of a technical society. On the other hand, the right hemisphere is good at achieving a sense of the whole. Whether we are dealing with the aesthetic sense of wholeness in a

poem or prayer, the grasp of the structural completeness of an inspiring tune, or the knowledge of the way a graphic design hangs
together as a whole, we are dealing with the reach for the larger
understanding. We may think of this as intuitive because the
simultaneous grasp of the whole is so complex that we have difficulty
explaining it in words.

It is likely that the detailing skills of the left hemisphere evolved
partly to record the flow of action in the world. Through language
we can tell a story without having to act it out. We can tell another
person how to do something without demonstrating every step.
Through music notation, we can recreate the sequence of a song.
Through a sequence of precise drawing steps, a conventionally
understandable design can be created. In a sense, detailed conventions can be used for helping us arrive at a whole. A drawing may be
grasped as a gestalt when it is finished, but it is created through one
sequence of actions or another. Conventionally laid-out sequences
are one means that allow people to learn from each other and arrive
at a technically manageable world.

However, the gestalt at its best is not quite what it is made out to
be in the conventionally understood sequence. You can instruct a
person on how to dance the waltz by telling the steps in the dance,
and this helps in learning. This is the very clumsy beginning of
dancing. Beyond this, there is a point when a person really begins to
do the waltz, and if he is good, a new dimension begins to enter.
There is a flowing wholeness to the dancing that can hardly be explained in the way that the rudiments were explained. The same
thing happens when a musician plays music. The first time through
the new music score, it sounds awkward and rigid. After the musician has played the score several times and moved beyond focus on
the individual notes, if the piece is done well, the musician grasps
the gestalt that the composer felt in creating the score, and the performance becomes inspiring.

The connections between skills involving sequential details and
those involving grasp of a gestalt are so intertwined that it is difficult
separating them when observing human activity. It is fair to assume
that most gifted children use both modes very well and relate the two
modes to each other with relative ease. There are human differences, however, and we need to have special concern for children
whose greatest strength is the grasp of complex structure. When

these children have difficulty using conventions of detailed sequencing, their special knowledge tends not to be recognized by others, and they are frustrated in using their specialized giftedness.

NEUROLOGICAL EXPLANATIONS

Attempts have been made to find neurologically based explanations for the distinct information processing in the two hemispheres. Jerre Levy-Agresti and Roger Sperry have suggested that the two kinds of processing may not be compatible in terms of the neuron organization required.[29] If this is true, it would provide a good evolutionary explanation for why the two kinds of processing were separated over time into the two hemispheres.

Josephine Semmes conducted research that hints at how this might work in the brain. Semmes studied sensory abilities in war veterans who had suffered localized brain injuries in either the right or left hemisphere. This involved testing the two hands for motor reactions, awareness of touch pressure in different locations, and discrimination between the location of sensations on the two hands. Testing of the right hand (left hemisphere) indicated a clear correspondence between skill deficiencies and the site of brain injuries, i.e. a particular skill deficiency could be consistently attributed to injury in a particular brain location. Testing of the left hand (right hemisphere) indicated much less precision in localization. Semmes suggested that the right hemisphere has a diffuse organization: "The proximity of unlike functional elements in a diffusely organized hemisphere would be expected to lead to a different type of integration from that characterizing a focally organized hemisphere; unlike units would more frequently converge, and therefore one might predict heteromodal integration to an extent surpassing that possible in a focally organized hemisphere."[30]

The diffuse organization of the right hemisphere might be advantageous for spatial tasks where a large amount of information needs to be synthesized all at once. It might, for example, allow a person to hold a geographic mapping of the United States in mind in an holistic way. Semmes is also suggesting that different kinds of experience can be brought together in this way. There can be a convergence of unlike elements such as visual, auditory, haptic, and proprioceptive information. All can be brought together in a single supramodal space. If this is true, it might account for the fact that

people who have difficulty speaking because of left hemisphere injury sometimes use metaphoric language in their attempts to communicate — language that often associates the various sensory
modes.

If the right hemisphere does specialize in integrating diverse
elements from our experience, it must possess an associational memory appropriate to the diversity. Metaphor is an associational process in which the most general physical qualities of things are used as
the basis of association. (The August day was a pressure cooker; the
child is a fish in water; the warrior is a lion.) In our ordinary
language, we tend to associate things by function: food words, trans-
portation words, movie titles, etc. In metaphoric language, the
association by general qualities opens up infinite possibilities.
(Name all the things that have at least one quality in common with a
hot August day.)

Jerre Levy-Agresti made other observations that would imply a
diffuse organization in the right hemisphere. She watched split-brain
patients as they explored three-dimensional objects with either their
left or right hand. Whereas the right hand would stop to focus on one
detail after another, the left hand would attempt to abstract the
gestalt of the object by immediately going over its surface as a whole.
Levy-Agresti suggests that "it was as if the speaking hemisphere processed stimulus information in such a way that the stimulus could be
described in language. Gestalt appreciation seemed to be actively
counteracted by a strong analytic propensity in the language hemisphere."[31] Similar observations have been made by Kimura and
Vanderwolf, and by Provins.[32]

IMPLICATIONS FOR THE EDUCATION
OF SPATIAL CHILDREN

The history of research on hemispheric asymmetry provides a
physiological foundation for expecting formal language abilities and
spatial understanding of gestalt structure to be independently represented in brain functioning. This research provides further credibili-
ty to the educator's observation that there are significant numbers of
children who are disproportionately capable in one or the other. It
should also lead educators to look for other skills and interests on the
part of children who are disproportionately strong in spatial ability,

e.g. an interest in expressive language such as poetry, and an appreciation for the more emotive qualities of music, which derive from a grasp of its holistic structure. In Chapter 6, we will also consider the connections between personality characteristics found in spatial ability research and cerebral asymmetry research.

Having considered Albert Einstein as a spatial child in Chapter 4, let us look briefly at some correspondences between his interests and the wider implications of asymmetry research. His spatial genius needs no comment. His slow development of language skills as a child was described in Chapter 4. Some difficulty with formal language continued throughout his life. When Einstein submitted his doctoral dissertation in 1905, one of his professors commented that in order to approve it, it was necessary to overlook certain "crudeness in style and slips of the pen."[33]

In spite of this continuing difficulty with formal language, Einstein was known to play around with expressive language throughout his life. He would often write little verses for his friends. For example, in 1930, while a colleague at Oxford University was away on a trip, Einstein stayed in his rooms and left this message for the absent host, Doctor Dundas.

Dundas lets his room decay
While he lingers far away,
Drinking wisdom at the source
Where the sun begins its course.

That his walls may not grow cold
He's installed a hermit old,
One that undeterredly preaches
What the Art of Numbers teaches

Shelves of towering folios
Meditate in solemn rows;
Find it strange that one can dwell
Here within their aid so well

Grumble: why's this creature staying
With his pipe and piano — playing?
Why should this barbarian roam?
Could he not have stopped at home?

Often, though, his thoughts will stray
To the owner far away,
Hoping one day face to face
To behold him in this place[34]

Einstein may never have succeeded as a poet, but he enjoyed this way of communicating as an alternative to more formal messages. Perhaps it is similar to Picasso who would seldom write letters. Instead, when he was away in Paris, Picasso would send cartoon messages to his parents.

Einstein had his own approach to music. He began taking violin lessons when he was six, but didn't enjoy learning because he was taught by rote rather than by inspiration.[35] Later he learned to play the piano. His appreciation increased after studying the mathematical structure of music. Mozart and Bach were two of his favorites. Although Einstein played music nearly all his life, he never became a particularly good performer. The precision and formality of perfected performance was not the thing that motivated him.

Einstein himself recognized the extent to which his appreciation for music derived from the same sources as his other mental processes. He once remarked that "music has no effect on research work, but both are born of the same source and complement each other through the satisfaction they bestow."[36] His eldest son observed that whenever Einstein "felt that he had come to the end of the road or into a difficult situation in his work, he would take refuge in music, and that would usually resolve all his difficulties."[37]

Those who are interested in the abilities of the right hemisphere should take interest in Einstein's collection of abilities and interests: unprecedented spatial understanding, enjoyment for creating poetry together with difficulties in formal language, and appreciation for the inspirational and structural qualities of music along with a disinclination for the finer, formal details of musical training and performance.

There is a growing sense among educators that the research on cerebral asymmetry has important implications for understanding varying learning styles among children and for understanding the needs of some children who have in the past been classified as learning disabled or underachievers. Jack Fadely and Virginia Hosler have been most ambitious in making these connections from their clinical observations on children. They describe some children as possessing "cerebral dissonance syndrome" or as being "alpha children." The term cerebral dissonance syndrome refers to an imbalance in the use of skills associated with the two hemispheres, an imbalance strongly favoring the skills of the right hemisphere. The meaning or need for the term alpha child is not so clear. Fadely and Hosler are interested in spatially skilled children who seem to possess a complex of other skills and attitudes associated with the right hemisphere — children who are, perhaps, the potential Einsteins and Picassos of their generation.[38]

There is one caution that educators should follow in using the terminology of cerebral asymmetry research. It is not possible to know the extent to which the behaviors of a child actually derive from right hemisphere processing. There are, for example, some people who have language functioning highly represented in both hemispheres. This can be so much the case that they can suffer serious left hemisphere injury and continue their verbal functioning at a highly proficient level. The incompatibility between the two kinds of thinking was suggested by Levy-Agresti and by Sperry. When formal language processes are highly represented in both hemispheres, it may result in some spatial deficiency. Spatial children (alpha children and genetic dyslexic children) may follow an opposite pattern in which spatial holistic skills are processed, to some extent, in both hemispheres. In this case the incompatibility results in a lowering of language efficiency in the left hemisphere.

As an example of these patterns, it is known that a certain portion of left-handed people have a poor separation of skills between the two hemispheres. In some of these left handers, this results in lower levels of spatial ability.[39] In the face of strong pressure toward becoming verbally competent people, these poorly lateralized left handers have suppressed spatial ability in favor of formal language. This can be true of those who pursue academic careers like the left-handed graduate students studied by Jerre Levy-Agresti.[40] Other left-handed people are known to be unusually competent in spatial ability. It is possible that under these conditions of incompatability and poor lateralization, this second group has gone in the direction of emphasizing spatial ability in both hemispheres.[41]

The principal point here is that brain functioning can follow a variety of patterns. Some spatial children may be processing spatial information in both hemispheres. Bannatyne strongly suggests that this is the case as pointed out in Chapter 3. It is important to remember this when using terminology that suggests that a child is predominantly right-brained in thought processes. We need to remain aware that this might not be the case in actual physical terms.

We use the terminology because in the average person this type of thought process is associated with the right hemisphere. The actual physical left-right association might not hold true in many spatial children.

In our efforts to recognize the virtues of right hemisphere thinking for the sake of spatial children, we need to observe one other caution. The prototype of a child who uses right hemisphere thinking almost exclusively could very well be the autistic child. In the descriptive work on the autistic child, one gets the impression of a child who has a natural inclination toward unusual spatial ability but no way to improve on this natural inheritance. The child has no way to make socially useful contributions because of an inability to relate to other people or to the accumulation of technical traditions in the society. We have no basis for describing what a proper balance might be between right hemisphere and left hemisphere thinking. A person like Albert Einstein might have leaned in the right hemisphere direction, but he certainly had enough balance between the two so that he could take good social advantage of his peculiar set of capacities.

Perhaps the most common situation is for people to use their right hemisphere processes for some of their more recreational activities, such as drawing, dancing, swimming, singing, and humor appreciation. They fail to apply the knowledge that can be derived from this experience to their intellectual processes. The Einsteins and Newtons are unusual in this regard. How many people would have seen an apple falling from a tree as being of any special intellectual significance? How do we arrive at a proper balance and relationship between naturalistic sensitivity and intellectual formality? We educators and psychologists are not very close to being able to answer this question with any precision.

Considering our lack of knowledge about varying patterns of brain functioning and our lack of knowledge about the balanced use of the thinking associated with the two hemispheres, it is best that we emphasize the things we do know with some confidence. We do know that certain kinds of intellectual processes seem to be compatible with each other in that they derive from similar cerebral organization. This knowledge allows us to look for certain skills and interests to cluster in certain children. This provides a well-founded basis for diagnosis and programming.

In any process of identifying spatial children, the primary piece of information to be looked for is a tendency for spatial skills to be stronger than language skills. Methods for doing this will be suggested in Chapter 7. Beyond this initial difference, it is sometimes the case that these children will have an appreciation for expressive aspects of language and music. Other personality differences will be explored in the next chapter.

REFERENCES

1. Taylor, J. *Selected Writings of John Hughlings Jackson.* New York: Basic Books, 1958, p. 148.
2. Harris, L.J. Neurophysiological factors in the development of spatial skills. In Eliot, J., and Salkind, N.J. *Children's Spatial Development.* Springfield, Ill.: Charles C Thomas, Publisher, 1975, pp. 7-8.
3. *Ibid.,* pp. 8-9.
4. Vygotsky, L.S. *Thought and Language.* Cambridge, Mass: M.I.T. Press, 1962.
5. Gazzaniga, M.S. The split brain in man. *Scientific American, 217:*24, 1967.
6. *Ibid.,* p. 25.
7. *Ibid.,* p. 27.
8. Durnford, N. Right hemisphere specialization for depth perception reflected in visual field differences. *Nature, 231:*394-395, 1971.
9. Kimura, D. Cerebral dominance and the perception of verbal stimuli. *Canadian Journal of Psychology, 15:*166-171, 1961.
10. Knox, C., and Kimura, D. Cerebral processing of nonverbal sounds in boys and girls. *Neuropsychologia, 8:*227-238, 1970.
11. Smith, J.M. Which hand is the eye of the blind? *Genetic Psychology Monographs, 5:*213-252, 1929.
12. Hermelin, B., and O'Connor, N. Functional asymmetry in the reading of braille. *Neuropsychologia, 9:*431-435, 1971.
13. Kimura, D. Spatial localization in left and right visual fields. *Canadian Journal of Psychology, 23:*445-458, 1969.
14. Witelson, S.F. Hemispheric specialization for linguistic and nonlinguistic tactile perception using a dichotomous stimulation technique. *Cortex, 10:*3-17, 1974.
15. Ingram, D. *Motor Asymmetries in Young Children.* University of Western Ontario Research Bulletin, 1973.
16. Bogen, J.E. The other side of the brain. In Ornstein, R. *The Nature of Human Consciousness.* New York: Viking Press, 1973, p. 108.
17. Bogen, *op. cit.,* p. 107.
18. Bogen, *op. cit.,* p. 108.
19. Bogen, *op. cit.,* p. 104.
20. Bogen, *op. cit.,* p. 104.
21. Bogen, *op. cit.,* p. 105.
22. Bogen, *op. cit.,* p. 105.

23. Kimura, D. Left-right differences in the perception of melodies. *Quarterly Journal of Experimental Psychology, 16:*355-358, 1964; Shankweiler, D. Effects of temperal lobe damage on perception of dichotically presented melodies. *Journal of Comparative Physiological Psychology, 62:*115-119, 1966.

24. Bogen, *op. cit.,* p. 106.

25. Bogen, *op. cit.,* p. 104.

26. Gardner, H. Composing symphonies and dinner parties. *Psychology Today, 13:*18, April 1980.

27. Gazzaniga, *op. cit.,* pp. 27-28.

28. Smith, I.M. *Spatial Ability: Its Educational and Social Significance.* London: University of London Press, 1964, pp. 96-97.

29. Levy-Agresti, J., and Sperry, R. Differential perceptual capacities in major and minor hemispheres. *Proceedings of the National Academy of Science, 61:*1151, 1968.

30. Semmes, J. Hemispheric specialization. *Neuropsychologia, 6:*11-26, 1968.

31. Levy, J. Possible basis for the evolution of lateral specialization of the human brain. *Nature, 224:*614-615, 1969.

32. Kimura, D., and Vanderwolf, C.H. Relation between hand preference and the performance of individual finger movement by left and right hands. *Brain, 93:*769-774, 1970; Provins, K.A. Handedness and skill. *Quarterly Journal of Experimental Psychology, 8:*79-95, 1956.

33. Clark, R.W. *Einstein: The Life and Times.* New York: Avon Books, 1971, p. 73.

34. *The London Times,* May 17, 1955. Translated by J.B. Leishman.

35. Clark, *op. cit.,* p. 29.

36. Clark, *op. cit.,* p. 141.

37. Clark, *op. cit.,* p. 141.

38. Fadely, J.L., and Hosler, V.N. *Understanding the Alpha Child at Home and School.* Springfield, Ill.: Charles C Thomas, Publisher, 1979, pp. 44-46.

39. *Ibid.,* pp. 62-63.

40. Fagan-Dubin, L. Lateral dominance and development of cerebral specialization. *Cortex, 10:*69-74, 1974.

41. Smith, I.M., *op. cit.,* p. 201.

Chapter 6

THE EXPANSIVE PERSONALITY

IT is commonly observed that people with distinct kinds of interests and abilities often seem to have personality characteristics that accompany their mental inclinations. Most people would own up to an intuitive sense that students who specialize in literature or theatre are in some sense different from those who specialize in mechanical drawing or mathematics. But the further contention that personality differences among children may indicate special needs within educational settings is less often thought about. It could be said that most teachers are given very little guidance on the special psychological needs of different groups of children. It is imperative that we explore personality research in relation to spatially gifted children, because their personality and character is often central to their approach to life, and acceptance of this fact is important in encouraging their intellectual development.

Research on the personality of the spatially-mechanically inclined person has a long and instructive history. In the 1920s, Max Freyd carried out an extensive set of studies in which spatially inclined people were compared to others. For his spatial group he selected 127 successful engineering students at the Carnegie Institute of Technology and the Case School of Applied Sciences. In order to have a comparison group of socially-verbally inclined people, he also studied 493 people who were either practicing salesman or students of salesmanship at the Carnegie Institute. He set up the groups in such a way that they would have an equal average IQ of about 110. In this way, he could assert that any differences found between the two groups were not caused by differences in intellectual ability.

Freyd created a questionnaire that had pairs of opposing personality descriptions. For example one opposing pair raised the possibility that a person could be either "absent-minded, continually absorbed in thought" or "wide-awake and alive to the present situation." Each engineering student and salesman was asked to indicate the extent to which one description or the other was appropriate for

125

their own personality. The two groups weren't always very different in the way they described themselves. However the direction in which each group leaned was very consistent and in line with the expectations of common wisdom. The two groups were at least a little different from each other on all items, and the differences were in the following directions[1]:

Engineers	Salesmen
Very absent-minded. Continually absorbed in thought.	Always wide-awake and alive to present situation.
Very ill natured and uncivil.	Very good-natured. Agreeable. Has winning manner.
Very slovenly and unkempt.	Extremely neat and clean. Almost a dude.
Always cool-headed and collected.	Very excitable and highstrung.
Extremely wary and hesitant. Acts only after careful consideration.	Always acts on the spur of the moment.
Considers himself incapable of much success.	Judges himself capable of anything.
Unimpressive physique and bearing.	Excites admiration. Very impressive.
Hidebound. Runs in a rut.	Is always adapting himself and taking up new ideas.
Lives almost entirely by himself.	Makes friends quickly and easily. Very popular.

If some of the descriptions of the spatially inclined engineers were not just extreme marker points toward which they were inclined more than the salesman, one could say the engineers were psychiatrically withdrawn. Few were so totally asocial. Freyd concluded, however, that the engineers were "self-conscious, careful of details, inhibited and cautious, reticent, absent-minded, and glum." The salesmen were described as having "social ability, credulity or suggestibility, adaptability, excitability, self-confidence, talkativeness, present-mindedness, and good-nature."[2]

Even in 1924 when Freyd published these results, there was already a long tradition of theorizing upon which to interpret them. In the late 1800s, William James had distinguished between the "explosive will" and the "obstructed will." In people with explosive will, "impulses seem to discharge so promptly into movements that inhibitions get no time to arise. Persons of that type are animated and talkative, and are possessed of great social abilities." Persons with obstructed will, on the other hand, are "more given to thought, they inhibit their reactions in order to allow thought to take place, but carry it too far. They are, at times, given to day dreaming."[3] In 1902, Baldwin made a similar distinction between a "sensory" type who looks inward and a "motor" type who acts outward.[4]

But it was Carl Jung who achieved the greatest influence on the theorizing about this distinction when he wrote about the "introvert" and the "extrovert."[5] Since the distinction comes up continually in the research related to spatially gifted people, Jung's definitions of these terms should be made clear. The emotions of the extrovert flow easily out into expression and action.

> They come in contact with life eagerly, spontaneously, without preparation or plan. If they show any timidity at all, the slightest encouragement has an immense effect upon them. They are that large group of people who are sociable and who accept social values unquestioningly. They are fond of amusement and are not greatly burdened by the problems of this world. They flow out into action and into emotional contact very easily; they express sympathy, delight, sorrow, appreciation, disgust, indignation, and jealousy without any difficulty. There is plenty of emotional play about their facial expressions and gestures when they are talking. They love movement, bustle, and excitement, and respond to what is going on around them with great facility. Studied closely, it is possible to see that between their feelings and the expression of these feelings there is little or no barrier.[6]

The introvert, on the other hand, is slow and reserved in the expression of emotion.

> The introvert type, in its most characteristic expression, is reserved, outwardly cold, guarded, watchful and difficult to understand. Unlike the extrovert, who hides little, the introvert hides everything because he dreads the exposure of his emotions, because they are too raw and intense. . . . He is thoroughly aware of his inner life, and is a keen and serious critic of himself. His tendencies lie in the direction of self-depreciation, which he often counterbalances by an outer air of self-appreciation. His approach to everything is critical and suspicious. . . . Anxiety is a constant state of mind with him; he is anxious about the future and anxious about the present. Fear is the predominant factor behind his psychology.[7]

When these two personality types suffer emotional difficulties, the symptoms of their stress form distinct patterns that have come to be the foundation of many classification theories of psychopathology. Extroverts become hysterics. Aspects of their mental lives are separated from each other in order to reduce stress. In dramatic cases, this can involve a loss of memory for some distinct period of time or the splitting of personality into separate, independent characters. Other times hysteria can involve a psychosomatic disability in which the form of the disability is a clue to the source of stress. During these difficulties, the hysteric remains a relatively cheerful, social being. Stress is handled through mentally partitioning the source of difficulty so that it doesn't have to be directly faced.

The introvert who is faced with undue stress tends to withdraw into an inner, morbid world. He is absorbed in internal conflicts, dead to the world, languid, self-centered, and full of free-floating anguish. Perhaps because he is the more internally aware of the two types, he is unable to adjust, as the hysteric does, by splitting his mental life.[8]

Two years after the publication of Freyd's research on engineers and salesmen, Ruth Hubbard reported a similar study on more than one thousand students at the University of Minnesota.[9] In her study, law students were used to represent the more socially-verbally inclined person, whereas engineering students were again used to represent the mechanically-spatially inclined. As expected, the engineers tended toward introversion and the law students leaned toward extroversion.

Anne Roe carried on in this tradition of relating personality variables to occupational status when she interviewed 22 prominent physicists in the early 1950s.[10] The physicists, as one might expect, scored exceptionally high on a spatial ability test; much higher than comparison groups of biologists, psychologists, and anthropologists. In comparison to these other groups, Roe also found the physicists to be unsociable and rather independent of social relations in general.

These studies of Freyd, Hubbard, and Roe on differences between occupational groups were fascinating and suggestive. But at the same time, other researchers were investigating the more direct relationship between ability test scores and personality measures. Himmelweit collected such test data in the 1940s and derived from it the spatial-verbal (k/v) factor discussed in Chapter 3.[11] One of the personality measures in that data was a measure of sociability. The verbal pole of the k/v factor was found to be associated with higher scores on the sociability measure, and the spatial pole was associated with lower sociability.

A few years later, Lewis Thurstone conducted a similar study.[12] In this study of ability factors, Thurstone found that mechanical ability correlated positively with the personality qualities that he called vigorousness and reflectivity. Mechanical ability correlated negatively with sociability. This combination of reflectivity with asocial attitudes is certainly consistent with Freyd's introversion findings.

THE NEGATIVE SIDE OF INTROVERSION

During the 1930s a more negative emphasis entered some of these personality investigations. One could already sense the unpleasant possibilities in the introversion as assessed by Freyd. A study by Uhler focused on these negative possibilities.[13] In a review of the school records of 820 children, Uhler found that children whose nonverbal test scores were superior to their verbal test scores were more frequently involved in delinquent and aggressive activities. In interpreting Uhler's findings, it might be asserted that delinquency and aggression are quite unlike introversion. The introvert might be unsociable, but he isn't usually thought of as being inclined toward actively hostile behavior. Nevertheless, the two are types of behavior that tend in the same asocial direction.

Perhaps when children who are relatively nonverbal and introverted experience frustrations, they are likely to react with aggressively hostile behavior. Not having the verbal means to express their anger or to manipulate other people, they respond in a nonverbal manner. This research result has led to a tradition in clinical psychology in which diagnosticians look for an ability pattern in which nonverbal test scores are significantly superior to verbal test scores. This is thought to provide the explanation for antisocial or even sociopathic behavior. In other words, if a child is more oriented toward manipulating objects than toward verbal relations with other people, then perhaps he will have a tendency to think of people as inanimate objects and treat them accordingly.

Considerable caution must be exercised in dealing with such assumptions. Clinical psychologists come into contact with large numbers of people who are disturbed in thought and behavior. Their diagnostic classifications are useful in understanding this minority of people. But it is totally unacceptable to apply their very imprecise testing procedures to the wider population. When people whose nonverbal intelligence is superior to their verbal intelligence become disturbed, they may tend in a sociopathic direction. Their nonverbal nature may channel the disturbance that way. The nonverbal nature, however, is not the cause of the disturbance.

It is important to protect the introverted, thoughtful approach to life as an acceptable version of normalcy. If we don't, the most natural inclination of a large group of children will be defined as abnormal, and this definition will become a source of low self-esteem for the children. Thoughtful self-sufficiency is a version of normalcy and should never become a characteristic for which a child must apologize. Unfortunately, in the verbal world of the school, too many children are made to feel inadequate because of this most natural inclination.

The other source of negative implications for the introverted personality comes from research on autistic children. Autism represents the extreme in asocial behavior. In the diagnosis of autism, asocial behavior combined with spatial ability is the key. In Kanner's classic attempt to establish diagnostic guidelines, two of his five criteria involve asocial tendencies.[14]

1. A profound lack of affective contact with other people.
2. Mutism, or a kind of language that does not seem to be intended to serve interpersonal communication.

Two of the remaining three criteria stress spatial-mechanical ability.

3. A fascination for objects, which are handled with skill in fine motor movements.
4. The retention of an intelligent and pensive physiognomy and good cognitive potential, manifested . . . by their skill on performance tests, especially the Seguin form board (a spatial test).

Kanner's only criterion not relating to either asocial character or spatial ability is the desire in the autistic child for the preservation of sameness in the environment. Autistic children often become disturbed when any object is not in its accustomed place. Even this might involve a need in these children to organize a consistent spatial gestalt in their minds.

During the past thirty years, various psychologists have suggested that autism represents an extreme position in a particular personality type and that there are many people who lean in this direction without extensive disabilities. Burns may have been the first to suggest this.

There is the type of case now known as "infantile autism," starting in infancy where speech is almost absent and there is a very marked lack of relationship to persons, while there is an obsessional interest in objects, particularly of a mechanical nature. Some of these children, while not completely autistic . . . grow up into the very eccentric type of individual, who never fits into society, but manages to live with fair success in a more or less private world.[15]

The personality of the spatially specialized child may simply represent the less extreme case of the autistically inclined person.

SHIFTING TERMINOLOGY AND EMPHASIS

Although the research that focused on the introversion-extroversion distinction may have seemed adequate for general purposes, personality study soon led to a refining of concepts. In the 1930s, Raymond Cattell succeeded in separating two aspects of personality that are closely related to the extroversion-introversion variable but yet distinct from it.[16] One of these he called the "surgency-desurgency variable" and the other he called the "cyclothymia-schizothymia variable." For many personality researchers from the 1950s to the present time, one or the other of these two variables has been the focus of attention in efforts to understand the spatially specialized personality. Whatever the slightness of distinction between these variables, it is of some value to become familiar with the distinctions.

Surgency-desurgency has to do with the flow of social energies. When Raymond Cattell was creating items for his personality questionnaires, he listed the following sets of opposing characteristics as being associated with surgency and desurgency.[17]

Surgency	*Desurgency*
Cheerful, joyous	Depressed, pessimistic
Sociable, responsive	Seclusive, retiring
Energetic, rapid in movement	Subdued, languid
Humorous, witty	Dull, phlegmatic
Talkative	Taciturn, introspective
Placid, content	Worrying, anxious
Resourceful, original	Slow to accept a situation
Adaptable	Bound by habit, rigid
Showing equanimity	Unstable mood level
Trustful, sympathetic, open	Suspicious, brooding, narrow

These characteristics emphasize the flow, or lack of flow, of social energies. Hebron used the surgency-desurgency variable to study personality patterns in a group of high school students.[18] From a group of 1,500 students, he selected seventy-six who had spatial test scores that were distinctly superior to their verbal test scores. Another group of fifty-six students had the opposite pattern. As expected, Hebron found that the spatial students tended toward desurgency, while the more verbal students tended toward surgency. Hebron also found that the spatial group was more independent, self-confident, and perseverant.

French arrived at similar results in a study reported a few years later.[19] After administering two spatial tests to groups of college students, he found that the students with higher spatial scores were more desurgent, less social, more nervous, and more emotional than other students. They were also more self-sufficient and self-confident. From both the Hebron study and the French study, we see the same pattern of introverted self-sufficiency observed by Freyd thirty years earlier in his engineering students.

Other researchers had a preference for the cyclothymia-schizothymia variable. These terms derived from Kretschmer in his studies of the personalities of men of genius in the 1920s.[20] Cattell managed to turn this into a measurable variable just as he had done with surgency-desurgency. In a similar manner, he began by listing the qualities.[21]

Cyclothymia	*Schizothymia*
Easy going	Obstructive, cantankerous
Adaptable	Inflexible, rigid
Warmhearted	Cool, indifferent
Frank, placid	Close-mouthed, secretive
Emotional, expressive	Reserved
Trustful, credulous	Suspicious, canny
Impulsive, generous	Close, cautious
Subject to emotional appeals	Impersonal
Humorous	Dry, impassive

Whereas the surgency-desurgency distinction emphasized the flow of social energies, the cyclothymia-schizothymia distinction seems to emphasize pro-social or antisocial feelings. Kretschmer, in his original use of the terms, had determined that some men of genius were characterized by schizothymia, particularly those in the sciences. Others were inclined toward cyclothymia, particularly those possessing literary genius. Pemberton, in the 1950s, and

Smith, in the 1960s, preferred to return to Kretschmer's concepts in their research.[22] They seemed to be drawn toward Kretschmer's position because of his connected theory on the relationship between personality and the thought processes that are crucial to spatial genius. We will return to that theory later in this chapter. A summary of the slight distinctions in the terminology employed by the various researchers is ventured in Table 6-I.

Table 6-I

Three Closely Related Variables that Have Been
Emphasized in the Study of the Relationship
Between Personality and Spatial Ability

Variable	Central Distinction
Extroversion vs. introversion	Degree of internal or external focus of attention
Surgency vs. desurgency	Extent of active flow of social energy
Cyclothymia vs. schizothymia	Extent of antisocial or pro-social feeling

In spite of the years since Freyd's original research report in 1924, and the many variations on the theme since then, his extroversion-introversion terminology still seems to be central to understanding the personality of the spatially specialized person. The qualities that have consistently gone along with introversion are self-confidence, independence, and self-sufficiency. When these characteristics are looked at together, a pattern appears in which an independence of thought is protected by a reluctance in relating the thoughts to other people. The person avoids pressure to accept superficial versions of conventional wisdom that lead away from piecing wisdom together as he himself encounters it. The spatially gifted person is often capable of a broad expanse of thinking. In this there is an attempt to relate a range of facts to each other in such a way that the patterns in the relationships are completely understood. The results of this expansive thinking cannot be easily related to others, nor can it be accomplished under conditions of social distraction.

The personality characteristics involve an insistence by the person on internal control of one's thoughts and feelings as a key feature in the independent mapping of the world. The introversion and independence in the spatially gifted person go together as a somewhat necessary underpinning for the mental work. At times, the introversion may go to the extreme of active avoidance of other people as in desurgency or to the extreme of strong antisocial feelings as in schizothymia. It could be hypothesized that these more extreme positions occur primarily when the spatially gifted person feels that his need for independent thought is under threat. Extensive desurgency and schizothymia could be seen as negative deviations from what otherwise would be a normal form of personal adjustment. It might also be hypothesized that a strong schizothymic reaction might have been more prominent in past centuries when there were more religious and doctrinaire pressures toward conformity of thought.

The inclination of men of scientific genius to become confirmed recluses may, at least in Western society, tend to be a relic of the past. Under past conditions, the thought processes of these men left them little choice but to withdraw from others if they were to be true to themselves. A healthy, independent introversion is probably the more normal form of this approach to life, and hopefully the more common approach today.

Although we may be improving in our allowance for independence of thought, we cannot say that this is no longer a problem in our schools. Independence of thought and investigation is not one of the more prominent qualities of most schools. There is no good reason to think that some of the men of genius of the past would today be much less pressed by the need to withdraw into themselves in order to pursue their creative activity.

ACCEPTING THE NEGATIVES OF PERSONALITY

This history of research on the personality of the spatially gifted person paints a rather negative picture. They are absent-minded, absorbed in thought, ill-natured, uncivil, slovenly, unkempt, cold, wary, hesitant, cautious, self-depreciating, unimpressive in physique, moody, hidebound, seclusive, secretive, taciturn, sluggish, depressed, pessimistic, retiring, subdued, languid, dull, phlegmatic, worrying, anxious, recalcitrant, rigid, suspicious, brooding, narrow, obstructive, cantankerous, canny, hostile, egotistical, impersonal, dry, and/or impassive. How could one compile a more negative cluster of human characteristics? If it couldn't be said that these characteristics reflect only the extreme end points toward which these people are inclined, and that few people actually reach the extreme, the picture might look horrendous. If we couldn't laud spatially competent people for their independence and self-sufficiency, we would have little good to say about them. If also we couldn't speculate that some of the characteristics are the result of reactions to unnecessary suppression of independent thought, the situation would seem hopeless.

Yet, it would not do to play down these characteristics as some educators have chosen to do. Some researchers on giftedness have attempted to establish a conventional wisdom that gifted children are generally better socially adapted than other people. This position has evolved from research on Lewis Terman's Stanford-Binet intelligence test. The Stanford-Binet is a highly verbal test, and no one would dispute the Terman conclusion that people who score high on the test tend to be socially well adjusted. However, the conclusion from the more general biographical research on people of significant accomplishment as carried out by Lombroso, Kretschmer, Barron, Roe, and Smith is quite different.[23] From the beginning of this line of study, it has been clear that significant amounts of social maladaption is found among people of creative accomplishment. It is an act of intellectual distortion to pretend, on the basis of the Terman research, that this is not true. It may allow a candy-coated approach to the understanding of gifted children, but it won't prepare us for the real characteristics encountered in many gifted children. If we are to understand the needs of gifted children, we must see the world as it is, even the personality characteristics of the spatially gifted child.

CONNECTIONS TO THE CREATIVE PERSONALITY

Research has tended to establish a connection between spatial ability and creativity. Drake and Schnall assessed creative potential in a group of learning-disabled children.[24] These children were selected for having mechanical abilities that were clearly superior to their language abilities and general school performance. Drake and Schnall gave the children sets of colored toothpicks and asked them to create as many different designs as they could with the toothpicks. These disabled children created a significantly greater number of designs than a comparison group of nondisabled children. This toothpick activity gives a measure of ideational fluency. In other words, when given a problem with no one correct answer, how many ideas can a child generate that could be solutions to the problem? Ideational fluency is known to be one basis for creative production. It should also be noted that the creative activity was of a spatial nature appropriate to the children. It is likely that if the activity had been of a different kind, such as theatrical improvision, the results would have been quite different.

A variety of theories are available for explaining why spatially competent children might have an inclination for certain kinds of creativity. Gestalt psychology is prominent among these theories, especially the theory of creativity provided by Konrad Lorenz. In Gestalt psychology, the capacity for form perception is central to higher levels of understanding and to problem solving. Form perception is important in the simple act of object recognition; however, it is equally important in recognizing patterns in information of all kinds. For Lorenz, creativity is the highest level of form perception in which some previously unseen pattern emerges from information; a discovered pattern that then becomes the basis for more adequate understanding of relationships in the gestalt. Lorenz writes —

> I hold that Gestalt perception of this type is identical with that mysterious function which is generally called intuition. . . . When the scientist, confronted with a multitude of irregular and apparently irreconcilable facts, suddenly "sees" the general regularity ruling them all, when the explanation of the hitherto inexplicable all "at once" jumps out at him with the suddenness of a revelation, the experience of this happening is fundamentally similar to that other when the hidden Gestalt in a puzzle-picture surprisingly stares out from the confusing background of irrelevant detail.[25]

Since the form perception in Gestalt psychology is virtually identical to the pattern recognition and transformation capacities central to spatial ability, the Lorenz theory would give good reason to expect spatially competent children to be highly creative in some ways.

Pemberton provided a slightly different explanation for the spatial ability-creativity connection.[26] Considerable research has indicated that a thinking quality called *flexibility of closure* is important in some forms of creative work. This quality involves resistance to arriving at quick, superficial conclusions. It facilitates the attempt to relate large amounts of information in terms of open possibilities. It allows careful shifting of focus from one aspect of information to another so that each aspect can be related to the whole. This requires slow, meticulous information processing. Flexibility of closure is thought to contrast with speed of closure, in which a person is attempting to process information in a fast and, of necessity, more superficial manner. Speed reading would be facilitated by speed of closure. Creating a logically connected outline for a writing project would be facilitated by flexibility of closure.

In his research, Pemberton administered a number of ability tests to 154 students. He used factor analysis to determine the ways these tests hung together and then studied the way the clusters of tests were associated with the temperamental qualities of students. The first factor corresponded to speed of closure, and the second to flexibility of closure. Pemberton noted that spatial tests were among those most heavily involved in the flexibility of closure factor. This included concealed figures, figure copying, figure classification, and designs. Pemberton found that the students who were high on flexibility of closure tended to be reflective, analytical, imaginative, and free of the need for social approval.

> The ability to detach the ego from the outer world, and the ability to account for acts to oneself are also characteristics of the abstract attitude. The lack of sociability and independence of social convention expressed by the subjects . . . suggest that these subjects do detach their egos from the outer world. . . . The dislike for routine and lack of tidiness . . . seems to stem from their flexibility, and not from impulsivity as their scores do not show any positive association with items dealing with impulsivity, and they say that they think of the consequences before acting. . . . High scores on reflectiveness and imagination also indicate the ability for thinking things over, and the tendency towards inner rather than outer orientation. However, the detachment of the . . . group from the outer world does not seem to be so complete as to be unrealistic, for they state that they are interested in achievement and recognition.[27]

Pemberton's research not only suggests a connection between creative imagination and spatial ability; it also arrives at the same introverted, self-sufficient personality that has come to be associated with spatial ability. This same personality cluster has come to be associated with the creatively productive person. In two successive studies, Drevdahl and Cattell found that creatively productive artists and scientists were more schizothymic, withdrawn, desurgent, and self-sufficient than groups of equally intelligent but less creative persons.[28]

The most extensive studies of highly creative people have been carried out by Frank Barron, Donald MacKinnon, and Ann Roe at the Institute of Personality-Assessment and Research at the University of California. They would invite writers, architects, artists, and scientists who were recognized by their colleagues for exceptional creative work to Berkeley for several days of intensive interviews. This would include filling out numerous personality inventories. There would be fireside chats with wine in the evenings. The creative people as a group were found to be preoccupied with ideas rather than people. They were poorly socialized, unconventional in the way they thought, uninfluenced by the opinions of others, and somewhat ungregarious. In addition, many personality strengths were found among the creative people. They were more flexible, curious, sensitive to their environments, and open to experience. They preferred complexity and were aware of their internal feelings, perseverant, sensitive to problems, and high in ego strength.

Looking at the antisocial and unconventional side of the behavior of these people, patterns were found that correspond closely to those of people suffering significant psychopathology. Looking at their strengths, the creative people could be seen as healthier, or at least much stronger, than the average person. Barron writes about these creative people:

> Psychometrically, such a pattern would be quite unusual. . . . Nevertheless, just such an unusual pattern is found. . . . If one is to take these test results seriously, creative individuals appear to be both sicker and healthier psychologically than people in general. Or, to put it another way, they are much more troubled psychologically, but they also have far greater resources with which to deal with their troubles. This gibes rather well with their social behavior, as a matter of fact. They are clearly effective people who handle themselves with pride and distinctiveness, but the face they turn to the world is sometimes one of pain, often of protest, sometimes of distance and withdrawal; and certainly they are emotional.[29]

Barron is most definitely following in the Lombroso and Kretschmer tradition of accepting the facts of both strength and social maladjustment in many gifted people. This is the tradition that many educators led by Lewis Terman have attempted to eliminate by equating high scores on the Stanford-Binet intelligence test with giftedness. They have, of course, ignored the fact that the Stanford-Binet has a very limited relationship with ultimate creative accomplishment. If we want to be ethically true to the responsibility of serving the broader population of gifted children, we must be ready to accept the nature of giftedness even when it offends our sense of conventionality. In the conclusion to one of his research reports, Frank Barron suggests that highly creative people are —

> As the common man has long suspected them to be, a bit "dotty." And of course it has always been a matter of pride in self-consciously artistic and intellectual circles to be, at the least, eccentric. "Mad as a hatter" is a term of high praise when applied to a person of marked intellectual endowments. But the "divine madness" that the Greeks considered a gift of the gods and an essential ingredient in the poet was not, like psychosis, something subtracted from normality; rather, it was something added. Genuine psychosis is stifling and imprisoning; the divine madness is a liberation from the consensus.[30]

To the extent that the spatial child exhibits unusual creativity, and to the extent that the personality characteristics of the spatial child are similar to those of the creative child, teachers and parents must be prepared to accept a degree of social unusualness in behavior.

CEREBRAL ASYMMETRY, CREATIVITY, AND PERSONALITY

In Chapter 5, it was suggested that there is a special relationship between creative behavior and right cerebral hemisphere functioning. The most dramatic evidence for this relationship comes from reports on creative people who have suffered disease or injury to their left hemisphere and yet retained much of their capacity for being creative in spite of other disabilities. Arieti has briefly reviewed a number of these cases.

> Luria, Tsvetkova, and Futer (1965) reported the case of a famous composer who, after a hemorrhage in the left temporal region, was unable to distinguish the sounds of speech or to understand words spoken to him, and yet continued "to compose brilliant musical works." Bonvicini (1926) reported the case of the painter Daniel Urrabieta (known under the name of Vierge) who, after cerebral apoplexy resulting in right hemiplegia, severe motor aphasia, and alexia, but no semantic aphasia, started to paint using the left hand and achieved such success that he became a

famous illustrator in the most important French periodicals. Alajouanine, too (1948), reported three patients who retained artistic creativity after they developed aphasia. Zaimov, Kitov, and Kolev (1969) reported the case of a Bulgarian painter who developed hemiplegia and aphasia as a result of cerebral apoplexy. This painter, famous before his illness, continued to paint afterwards with great success. As with Vierge, he used the left hand instead of the right; his painting also changed tonality, as light colors came to be used more frequently; and the compositions became less stylized. At the time of the report, sixteen years after the cerebral accident, the painter continued to work with great success and his paintings were highly appreciated.[31]

Research that attempts to establish the connection between right and left hemisphere functioning and creativity in persons without brain damage is being actively pursued, but is less convincing.[32] Sorting out the activities of the intact brain is perhaps the biggest challenge to psychologists, and understanding the nature of creative behavior runs a close second in difficulty. Unraveling the relationships between the two multiplies the complexities. One of the difficulties in this line of research is that there may be two rather distinct forms of creativity. One form may involve an uninhibited associational flow of the kind that could be valuable to a novelist or an improvising actor. The other kind of creativity may involve a mapping of relationships in a pattern or system. This second type might be more valuable to a scientist or a sculptor.

Prentky has suggested that the first type of creativity might derive primarily from the left hemisphere and the second type from the right.[33] To the extent that these two types of creativity are independent of each other, any research effort that has attempted to treat them as if they were identical would be misleading. Since I do not know of one research study on the relationship between creativity and cerebral asymmetry that makes this distinction, it is likely that the whole line of research on this topic is flawed.

Nevertheless, it is obvious from the more global observations on brain-damaged patients that there is a special relationship between right hemisphere function and certain forms of creativity. An obvious question that should be explored is whether the personality similarities found between people who are specialized for spatial ability and people who are noted for creative production might in some way derive from right hemisphere functioning. Might a right hemisphere dominance be responsible for the independent, introverted, desurgent, schizothymic personality type that is associated with spatial ability and observed among a large portion of highly creative people? A tradition of research in neuropsychology strongly suggests this possibility.

Robert Prentky has reviewed a number of neurological studies that suggest that weakness in the left hemisphere, and the implied domination of cognition by the right hemisphere, can result in schizophrenia and other symptoms of psychosis.[34] In some of this research, the weakness of the left hemisphere is the result of war injuries. In other studies it has been the result of tumors. This type of observation led Gruzelier and Hammond to suggest that schizophrenia occurs when left hemisphere processing is unable to keep up with the gestalt information processing of the right hemisphere.[35] This results in the overgeneralized, overinclusive thought processes that are characteristic of the schizophrenic. The opposite pattern of weakness in the right hemisphere, and domination by left hemisphere thinking, tends to lead to manic-depressive symptoms and other affective disturbances.

The point to be made here is that there are sound clinical reasons for suspecting that the introversion and schizothymia that characterize spatially gifted people, and a large portion of highly creative people, derive from the right hemisphere in the same way that their special abilities derive from that hemisphere. It is interesting that with these developments in neuropsychology, psychologists are led back to the same personality distinctions that Kretschmer proposed early in this century as being associated with creativity of different types.

A PHYSIOLOGICAL EXPLANATION

When MacFarlane Smith wrote his monumental work on spatial ability, he integrated a set of research findings that may provide an explanation for the relationship between abilities and personality characteristics. Basic to the explanation is the idea that spatial ability requires the capacity to hold a complicated system of interconnected information in mind and the capacity to manipulate that information in such a way that none of the relationships in the system are ever violated. This would be true of an architect creating a plan for a building. Every detail in the whole must hang together in some logical way. This requires having this information remain unconfused by irrelevant external information. Thus, there is the need for a degree of introversion.

In support of this position, Smith cites research by Mundy-Castle that indicates that spatially capable people tend to have a higher degree of cortical arousal than other people.[36] The alpha index derived from electroencephalogram measures of brain activity is an indication of cortical relaxation. Mundy-Castle found that the alpha index is inversely related to spatial ability. This would indicate that while the spatially competent person is avoiding contact with the outside world through his introversion, a high level of mental activity is going on internally. The person is evidently avoiding confusion from external information in order to carry on active internal thought processes.

This description of the spatially capable person fits well with Eysenck's concept of reactive inhibition.[37] Eysenck suggests that retaining information in one's mind is an active process requiring an inhibition of external information. The energy required for this inhibition is continually accumulated and dissipated in a pattern characteristic of the individual personality and type of mental activity. An introverted person requires more of this inhibitory effect as a prerequisite to carrying on a more complex, internal mental life.

These concepts also fit well with the idea of a separation between people who have primary strength in verbal skills and those who have primary strength in spatial skills. Essential to verbal ability is the capacity to process many details in quick succession. Cyril Burt contends that when watching children read, two different styles tend to be observed. One type of child is slow and meticulous, hanging on every word. The other type of child is quick and more superficial. Burt called the slow, meticulous reader the fixating type. The quick reader he called the diffusive type. Burt describes the reading behavior of the two types.

> Faced with some unfamiliar object or pattern — say a sentence, to be read aloud, like "fair waved the golden corn" — one child will focus his glance fixedly on one little group of letters after another, uttering the whole in detached installments — "Fair,   wav -ed,   the   gold—en, corn." Another whose eye roves rapidly up and down the line, will produce some impressionistic version superficially corresponding to the general visible scheme, if not to the detailed parts — "A fairy waved her golden wand."[38]

The fixating child evidently has difficulty processing the details in the reading material and fitting them quickly into a mental gestalt. The diffusive child can evidently do this more quickly. We are reminded of Colin MacLeod's research on reading behavior reviewed in Chapter 3.[39] MacLeod found some people require a distinctly longer time to process reading information than is normal. The same people are much more efficient in using the information once it is processed. MacLeod's theory is that these slow readers are processing the information directly into a spatial mode. MacLeod's observations fit very well with Burt's observations. Like MacLeod, Burt found children who were stronger in spatial ability to be more often among the slower, fixating perceivers. Burt also found them to be introverted and to have a more self-sufficient and persistent character. Burt found children who were stronger in verbal skills to be more often among the quicker, fluctuating perceivers, to be more extroverted, and to be less self-sufficient and persistent in character. MacLeod's distinct slow readers were often among those highest in spatial ability.

Based on such observations, MacFarlane Smith concluded that a fixative attention, and a tense, selective inhibitive approach to experience are key to the mental process of the spatially specialized person. This is the explanation for the introverted, independent personality.

Smith explains this selective inhibition of experience in terms derived from the gestalt school of psychology. The process of integrating experience into wholes is accomplished in part by inhibiting the perception of unimportant or inconsistent details. In gestalt psychology this is called the law of *pragnanz*. The mind organizes the stimulus field into the best holistic pattern that experience will permit. For example a picture of a circle with a gap in it is seen as being a circle in spite of the gap. The mind perceives the best structure possible and accomplishes this by inhibiting perception of the unimportant details that fail to be consistent with the structure. "The exceptional ability of the spatially gifted person for perceiving structure or form may depend on a capacity for selective inhibition of experience and this may be a general characteristic of his whole personality."[40]

It would hardly be appropriate to demean the life-style of the spatially gifted person; a life-style that has lead to the invention of the calculus and the general theory of relativity; a life-style that has led to the painting of the *Guernica* and the construction of the *Burghers of Calais*. Yet, there are definitely some potential weaknesses in the personality style. Problems tend to arise when some source of tension leads the introverted person to begin overgeneralizing on the basis of some rigid, internal map of reality and to discontinue incorporating new information that might require adjustments in the map. The lack of relationship to external reality then leads to maladaptive thought processes and behavior. In 1947, Cameron compiled information that indicated that the disorganizing quality of the thought process in schizophrenia is the formation of overly large and vague concepts.[41] This has come to be a prominant diagnostic criterion in the identification of schizophrenia.

In talking about the potential for schizophrenia, it is important to insist that this is only an extreme point that few spatially gifted people ever reach. The capacity to interrelate large expanses of information is one of the valuable capacities of the spatially gifted child. As long as this generalizing capacity doesn't rigidify on untested conclusions that are disconnected from reality, it can be the basis for profound intellectual work.

PERSONALITY OF THE ALPHA CHILD

In their description of the alpha child, the ability indicators that Jack Fadely and Virginia Hosler mention are essentially the same as those characterizing the spatial child, i.e. spatial-mechanical test scores higher than verbal-academic scores.[42] It is therefore valuable to consider the described personality of the alpha child in relation to personality research. Fadely and Hosler described what they saw in their clinical observations on children without much reference to the past research. In this sense, they provide a valuable independent perspective.

Central to their understanding of the alpha child is *naturalistic cognitive function*. Since the alpha child approaches the world in an independent, global, poorly verbalized, and unsocialized manner, the child tends to see the physical world in a direct, natural way.

> Our naturalistic tendency in perception and cognitive function is to organize information into a "gestalt" or to see the entirety of a thing, a thought, or a feeling as opposed to looking at individual parts as in

socialized and evaluative thought. This naturalistic and total response tendency is most closely attuned to the senses such as smell, taste, touch, sound in the form of nonverbal or musical activity, and, most importantly feelings or emotion. Thoughts can come rushing in upon our naturalistic mind that are emotionally overwhelming, totally absorbing, and highly fulfilling. There are not words, we often say, to explain how we feel. This is the world of high psychic and mystical awareness. When we are totally in love, when a musical score brings ecstasy, when we come to feel a oneness with nature, or when we are suddenly aware of the meaning of God, these are naturalistic and highly sensory thoughts which exist beyond social evaluation and words. . . . Most importantly, for cognitive organization, we experience a thought process which deals primarily with total impression, space, and images of the moment.[43]

For Fadely and Hosler,* this naturalistic cognitive functioning is associated with the right hemisphere. Developmentally, they see this as predominating in most young children and usually it recedes with age. It is a person's first natural way of looking at the world. Gradually added to it is a more socialized view of the world that is organized in verbal categories and that has language to provide an organizing and mediating relationship to the world. Whereas naturalized thought processes are more present-oriented and devoid of time perspective, socialized thought emphasizes the significance of current behavior as a logical continuation of previous experience and as having logical implications for future events. Socialized behavior becomes goal-directed and consistent over time. The alpha child is seen as lagging behind others in adding this socialized perspective to the naturalized.

The positive side of this view is that the alpha child has an independent perspective on the world, unhampered by the formulations of others. This can result in greater creativity. The negative side is that the child is neither able to relate socially to other children or to learn from the accumulated knowledge of others. Not being able to relate to others in a socialized way, the child gets frustrated in social situations and may employ "fight or flight" acting-out behaviors. This description of the alpha child does fit quite well with the asocial behavior found in the research on spatial ability.

Fadely and Hosler provide a valuable clinical perspective. Some caution should be used, however, in interpreting their views. They

---

*From Jack Fadely and Virginia Hosler, *Understanding the Alpha Child at Home and School*, 1979. Courtesy of Charles C Thomas, Publisher, Springfield, Ill.

see the alpha child somewhat as suffering from a developmental lag. One gets the impression that the child didn't have the proper socializing experience and that if the proper experiences are provided, the pattern of behavior will change. This is somewhat different from the MacFarlane Smith position or the Alexander Bannatyne position, in which the spatially specialized child is seen as possessing an inherent cognitive style. The style shapes both intellectual work and social outlook. From the Smith and Bannatyne position, one can assist the social adjustment of the child, but the basic cognitive style is likely to remain for life, along with remnants of the introversion.

It is important to be cautious on this point because of the possible confusions that could be involved. There are many poorly socialized children in our schools, and spatial children may have a somewhat greater tendency than other children to be seen as poorly socialized. But to equate the two would be a mistake. A spatial child can have a perfectly adequate socialization experience and yet not be highly effective in social ways. Other children can be poorly socialized and yet not have a very adequate global, spatial understanding of the world around them. Sometimes spatial ability and poor socialization are present in the same child, but we should not assume a necessary connection between the two. It is one thing to be poorly socialized and another to have asocial inclinations in spite of socializing experiences.

Many spatially specialized children have probably had very positive socialization experiences. There are psychologists who think that the cognitive approach of the spatial child is sometimes the result of socialization. There is evidence that an unusual portion of children growing up in rural farm situations are stronger in spatial skills than verbal. This is thought to be the result of their need to develop strong practical and mechanical skills in order to participate in the way of life of their families. Their cognitive style is the result of good socialization, not poor socialization. Their cognitive style may also be accompanied by a less verbal and more introverted personality than that of their city cousins. This, too, is the result of socialization.

Along this same line of caution, it is important not to equate right hemisphere information processing with irrational, out-of-control thought processes. When the right hemisphere attempts to synthethesize large amounts of information into gestalt systems, the result may be difficult to communicate to others. It certainly seems highly intuitive, but not irrational. Anyone who has completed the space relations subtest from the Differential Aptitude Tests will verify that highly rational and highly systematic thought is required. Any child who has completed the block design subtest from the Wechsler Intelligence Scale for Children has carried out a rational act.

Here, as in other places, we must guard against equating verbal behavior with rationality. For too long educators have operated under the principle that if a child can't explain his ideas in words, the ideas probably aren't worthy of consideration. The architect who creates a blueprint for a building is carrying out a highly rational act, even though he communicates his ideas best through a graphic representation.

REFERENCES

1. Freyd, M. The personality of the socially and mechanically inclined. *Psychological Monographs, 33*:1-49, 1924.
2. *Ibid.,* p. v.
3. Freyd, M. Introverts and extroverts. *Psychological Review, 31*:74-87, 1924.
4. Baldwin, J.M. *The Story of the Mind.* New York: Appleton and Company, 1902.
5. Jung, C.G. *Analytic Psychology.* London: Bailliere, Tendall and Cox, 1916.
6. Nicoll, M. *Dream Psychology.* London: Hodder and Stoughton, 1921, p. 139.
7. *Ibid.,* p. 139.
8. McDougall, W. *Is America Safe for Democracy?* New York: Charles Scribner's Sons, 1921, p. 85.
9. Hubbard, R.M. Interests studied quantitatively: measurement of differences between the socially and mechanically inclined in relation to vocational selection. *Journal of Personnel Research, 4*:365-378, 1926.
10. Roe, A. A psychological study of eminent psychologists and anthropologists and a combination with biologists and physical scientists. *Psychological Monographs, Vol. 67,* 1953.
11. Himmelweit, H.T. The intelligence-vocabulary ratio as a measure of temperament. *Journal of Personality, 14:*93-105, 1945.
12. Thurstone, L.L. *An Analysis of Mechanical Aptitude.* Chicago: University of Chicago Psychometric Lab Report, No. 5, 1951.
13. Smith, I.M. *Spatial Ability: Its Educational and Social Significance.* London: University of London Press, 1964, p. 218.
14. Kanner, L. Problems of nosology and psychodynamics in early childhood autism. *American Journal of Orthopsychiatry, 19:*416, 1949.
15. Burns, C.L. Psychosis in children. *Quarterly Bulletin of the British Psychological Society, 10:*389-390, 1950.

16. Cattell, R.B. Temperament tests. *British Journal of Psychology, 24:*20-49, 1933.
17. Cattell, R.B. *Personality and Motivation.* Yonkers-on-Hudson, New York: World Book Company, 1957, p. 112.
18. Hebron, E.A. *Status of Pupils in Various Streams of Secondary Modern Schools.* University of Hull: Institute of Education Studies in Education, 1957, p. 5.
19. French, J.W. *Comparative Prediction of Success and Satisfaction in College Major Fields.* Princeton, N.J.: Educational Testing Service, 1959.
20. Kretschmer, E. *The Psychology of Men of Genius.* London: Kegan Paul, 1930.
21. Catell, *op. cit.,* 1957, p. 90.
22. Smith, *op. cit.,* p. 226; Pemberton, C.L. The closure factors related to temperament. *Journal of Personality, 21:*159-175, 1952.
23. Lombroso, C. *The Man of Genius.* London: Walter Scott, 1891; Barron, F. The psychology of creativity. In Rothenberg, A., and Hausman, C. *The Creativity Question.* Durham, N.C.: Duke University Press, 1976, pp. 196-197.
24. Drake, C. and Schnall, M. Decoding problems in reading. *Pathways in Child Guidance,* Vol. 8. 1966.
25. Lorenz, K.Z. The role of gestalt perception in animal and human behavior. In Whyte, L.L. *Symposium on Aspects of Form.* London: Lund Humphries, 1951.
26. Pemberton, *op. cit.,* pp. 159-175.
27. Pemberton, *op. cit.,* 159-175.
28. Drevdahl, J.E. *An Exploratory Study of Creativity in Terms of Its Relationship to Various Personality and Intellectual Factors.* Ph.D. thesis, University of Nebraska, 1954; Cattell, R.B., and Drevdahl, J.E. A comparison of the personality profile of eminent researchers with that of eminent teachers and administrators and of the general public. *British Journal of Psychology, 46:*248-261, 1955.
29. Barron, *op. cit.,* pp. 196-197.
30. Barron, *op. cit.,* p. 196.
31. Arieti, S. *Creativity: The Magic Synthesis.* New York: Basic Books, 1976, p. 399.
32. Prentky, R.A. *Creativity and Psychopathology.* New York: Praeger Publishers, 1980, pp. 116-117.
33. *Ibid.,* p. 129.
34. *Ibid.,* pp. 120-122.
35. Gruzelier, J., and Hammond, N. Schizophrenia: a dominant hemisphere temporal-lobe disorder? *Research Communications in Psychology, Psychiatry and Behavior, 1:*33-72, 1976.
36. Mundy-Castle, A.C. Electrophysiological correlates of intelligence. *Journal of Personality, 26:*184-199, 1958.
37. Eysenck, H.J. Cortical inhibition, figure after-effect, and the theory of personality. *Journal of Abnormal of Social Psychology, 51:*94-106, 1955.
38. Burt, C. The structure of the mind. *British Journal of Educational Psychology, 19:* 176-199, 1949.
39. MacLeod, C.M., Hunt, E.B., and Mathews, N.N. Individual differences in the verification of sentence-picture relationships. *Journal of Verbal Learning and Verbal Behavior, 17:*493-507, 1978.
40. Smith, *op. cit.,* p. 291.
41. Cameron, N. *The Psychology of Behaviour Disorders,* Boston: Houghton Mifflin,

1947.

42. Fadely, J.L., and Hosler, V.N. *Understanding the Alpha Child at Home and School.* Springfield, Ill.: Charles C Thomas, Publisher, 1979.

43. *Ibid.,* pp. 80-81.

SECTION II

WORKING WITH

THE SPATIAL CHILD

Chapter 7

IDENTIFYING SPATIAL CHILDREN

W HEN identifying spatial children in a school context, it is important to relate the identification procedures to the psychology of giftedness so that spatial children, when appropriate, can legitimately take their place in programs for the gifted. It is therefore important to work from a general understanding of giftedness and to make identification procedures, appropriate to spatial children, fit the general understanding. Two current research-based identification models have evolved from the work of Joseph Renzulli at the University of Connecticut and that of Abraham Tannenbaum at Columbia University.[1] I have merged aspects of both models to create my own model, which I call the significant accomplishment model.

The key difference between the Renzulli and Tannenbaum models in comparison to most traditional identification approaches is the directionality of the research that supports them. In most traditional conceptions, a specific psychometric test is administered to a group of children; then, at some later point in time, the accomplishments of the children are assessed. The relationship between the test scores and the later accomplishments then becomes the justification for the use of the test in subsequent identifications of gifted children. Most noted in this tradition is the work of Lewis Terman and E. Paul Torrance.

The Renzulli and Tannenbaum models tend to be justified by a reverse time directionality of research. In other words, highly accomplished adults are identified, and then the childhoods of these accomplished people are assessed to determine what childhood characteristics were common to these adults. These characteristics then become the basis for subsequent identification procedures. The difference in the two approaches can be seen in Figure 7-1.

The advantage of this second approach is that it can result in a much more developed understanding of the various components that enter into the realization of significant accomplishment. If the traditional psychometric approaches had proven powerful in terms of the prediction of ultimate accomplishment, they would most likely have

153

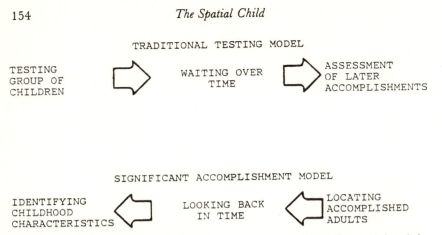

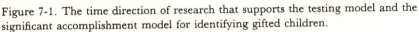

Figure 7-1. The time direction of research that supports the testing model and the significant accomplishment model for identifying gifted children.

retained their supremacy. Research has indicated that this is not the case, necessitating a shift toward significant accomplishment models.

The research that supports significant accomplishment models is highly involved, and this can lead to varying interpretations as is obvious from differences between the Renzulli model and the Tannenbaum model. From my own reading of the research, I arrive at the following five characteristics of children — each of which may serve as a clue of potential for significant accomplishment:

1. A strong, focused interest in an area of endeavor
2. Above-average abilities that are appropriate to the area of interest
3. The capacity for a flexible, creative thinking that is appropriate to the area of endeavor
4. The capacity for protracted activities in the area of endeavor
5. A strong sense of self-determination

This model can be diagrammed as in Figure 7-2.

A BRIEF RESEARCH SUMMARY
ON THE SIGNIFICANT ACCOMPLISHMENT MODEL

Strongly Focused Interest

If there is anything that comes through clearly in the biographical

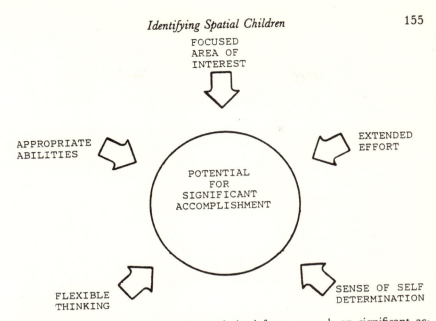

Figure 7-2. Components of giftedness derived from research on significant accomplishment.

literature on people of outstanding accomplishment, it is the intensity of their interest in their particular area of endeavor. In many cases, this intensity served to overcome weaknesses that threatened the opportunity to pursue the area of endeavor. This observation from biography is related to a variety of research studies on future career images conducted by Polak, Singer, Toffler, and Torrance.[2] In general, this research indicates that the more clearly children identify the future career areas they would like to pursue, the greater will be their adult accomplishments. Toffler claims that these career images are more predictive of future accomplishments than any past indicators of ability or accomplishment. Based on these findings, Torrance has suggested that it is important for teachers and parents to encourage children to "fall in love with something at an early age and investigate it in depth."[3]

The importance of this realization is that it puts the interests of children at a front and center position in the identification of giftedness. This is a difficult conclusion for traditional psychometricians to swallow, but, nevertheless, it seems to be an unavoidable conclusion.

Abilities Appropriate to Area of Interest

It also has become quite clear that most significant accomplishments are not based on some general intellectual capacity, but rather on capabilities that are appropriate to an area of interest. In relation to spatial ability, this conclusion has been reviewed in Chapters 2 and 3. In relation to social effectiveness, David McClelland has demonstrated that accomplishment in the leadership area does not derive so much from some general, vague intellectual ability as it does from certain specific skills appropriate to the area of social leadership.[4]

Considering the weight of the evidence accumulating in this area, it is surprising that those who are familiar with the literature remain attached to a general abilities model. For example, Joseph Renzulli still emphasizes the idea of general ability getting applied to specific areas of endeavor rather than looking first at the main area of interest and then verifying the existence of appropriate abilities.[5] Confusion on this point can mislead practitioners, preventing them from adjusting to the fact that children who possess potential for significant accomplishments in some areas of endeavor can at the same time possess significant weaknesses in other areas. In these cases, looking for general ability will tend to hide the potential that is there.

The neuropsychologist Reitan gives an interesting anecdote on the kind of misapplication of human ability that can result from failing to understand differences in human ability.[6]

> Some years ago, a resident neurological surgeon at the Indiana University Medical Center volunteered to take a battery of neuropsychological tests in order to have a better understanding of the types of examinations that might be given to his patients. After taking this extensive battery of psychological tests, that among other things yielded information concerning the differential status of the two cerebral hemispheres, he returned to obtain a brief interpretation of the results. The results indicated that this young neurosurgeon had an excellent left cerebral hemisphere, but that abilities dependent upon the right cerebral hemisphere were scarcely better than average. . . . The differential level of this man's abilities in these two areas prompted me to offer an initial comment to the effect that the test results indicated that he probably would be much better at telling about an operation after it was over than he would be at actually doing it. The neurosurgeon looked shocked, admitted that this was correct, and confessed that he regularly was the last person to be able to identify any landmarks! The test results, in other words, had definite practical implications with respect to the evaluation of the subject.

The surgeon was obviously a very talented person. Undoubtedly, he would never have reached this position in life had he not possessed considerable ability; so much linguistic ability that he was able to cover for his spatial deficiencies. Lack of knowledge of his own particular complex of abilities had led to his entering a field in which he was not particularly adept. On occasion, it might also have been of some danger to his patients. The general tendency in American society to think in terms of general ability rather than specific competencies has probably led to an unnecessary and wasteful amount of this misfitting.

The practical implication of this is that it doesn't do much good to assess the abilities of children until we know their areas of intense interest. Once areas of interest are known, it is possible to focus assessment on those skills that will be most crucial to accomplishment in the given area.

Creativity Appropriate to Area of Interest

The capacity to make unusual accomplishments in a given area often involves a flexibility in thinking, which allows the person to respond appropriately to new challenges rather than being stuck in old solutions to old problems. However, creative behavior takes a variety of forms, and we must be concerned that the kind of creativity we look for in a child is appropriate to the child's area of interest. Perhaps the most important distinction in creative thinking is that suggested by Prentky and mentioned in Chapter 6.[7] Some creativity relies heavily on ideational fluency of the kind that would be useful to an improvising actor. Other creativity relies more on gestalt transformations of the kind that would be useful to a scientist, a sculptor, or an architect.

Since most current tests of creativity stress ideational fluency, it is important to keep this distinction clearly in mind when looking for creative capacities in spatially inclined children. It is best to simply look for flexibility of thinking in their spatial production.

Capacity for Protracted Activities in the Area of Interest

Research has clearly demonstrated that those who realize the most outstanding accomplishments are most often those who have carried out a series of related activities over an extended period of time. This is part of what Joseph Renzulli means by task commitment.[8] Ann Roe has found that in many accomplished people, these activities started at a relatively early age.[9]

The potential problem in this area is the direction we look for evidence of relevant activities. It is too easy for *task commitment* to be defined as those behaviors that fit narrowly within the boundaries of some traditional academic performance. Since most outstanding accomplishment takes place outside of academic fields, it is important to have the widest possible view of task commitment. We educators must attempt to recognize any childhood behavior that could be a precursor to adult accomplishment. Had Isaac Newton's teachers recognized his construction of gadgets as an indication of his potential, he might have been seen as gifted rather than as learning-disabled. Had the childhood theatrical and journalistic activities of Winston Churchill been regarded as an indicator of potential, he might have been seen as gifted rather than hopeless. Had Isadora Duncan's dancing in the street outside of school been acknowledged for its creativity, her teachers might have seen her potential for being one of the greatest dancers of all time. Had his teachers appreciated his childhood speculations on the nature of magnetism, Albert Einstein might have been seen as a future scientist rather than as a failure.

One of the greatest challenges to educators of the gifted is achieving the openness of vision necessary for recognizing the precursors of genius. These stories of educator's blindness to giftedness will continue to accumulate as long as we continue to be shackled by narrow conceptions of giftedness. It is for this reason that we should be looking for protracted activities in the child's area of interest, and not just task commitment in some vague, usually academic sense.

Strong Sense of Self-Determination

Joseph Renzulli merges the idea of self-determination into the idea of task commitment. Certainly, they are closely related. But self-determination almost always is key to the passionate pursuit of interests among the truly gifted. Unless we focus on it as a separate issue, it would be too easy for task commitment to be defined in some regimented way.

When Charles Darwin was a school boy, he often got in trouble because of his divergent interests in chemistry and bug collecting. On one occasion, he was lectured by the headmaster in front of the student body at the Royal Free Grammar School of Shrewsbury. The headmaster said, "Darwin, you are wasting your time on useless subjects. Stick to your Greek grammar and Latin literature. They are the unfailing marks of an English gentleman."[10] Darwin did not take this advice. He went on pursuing his divergent studies. He once said about his years in college, "my best hours were spent in extracurricular activities but my professors were not interested in what I did outside their classrooms."[11] What Darwin did outside the classroom became the basis for his unique contribution to the world of ideas. Although he was a mediocre student at best, his strong sense of self-determination led to accomplishments beyond those of any of his peers.

Although it is sometimes difficult to accept the motivations toward self-determination in the school setting, research makes clear the extent to which it is an important aspect of most creative accomplishments.[12]

INFORMAL METHODS
FOR IDENTIFYING SPATIAL CHILDREN

The significant accomplishment model outlined above suggests that the identification of giftedness involves much more then looking for ability through some abstract testing method. Rather, the potential for giftedness must be seen in a complex pattern of interests, abilities, and motivations. A great deal of uncertainty must be accepted about this process as might be suggested by the fact that all psychometric approaches to predicting ultimate accomplishment have proven rather disappointing. This being the case, we should be somewhat liberal, as Abraham Tannenbaum suggests, in our screening procedures.

> Giftedness in children means different things to different people. But no matter what definition we accept, identifying it has to be counted among our inexact sciences, partly because the methods and instruments available for that purpose are imprecise. Besides, childhood is usually too early in life for talent to be fully-blown, so we have to settle for dealing

with talent-in-the-making and keep in mind the uncertainties about the future. Identification is, therefore, a matter of locating children who possess high potential in comparison to other children, with no guarantees that they will eventually excel by universal standards as adults, even with proper nurturance. In creating a pool of "hopefuls," it is best to admit any child who stands a ghost of a chance of someday making it to the top in the world of ideas. Of course, most "hopefuls" are really "doubtfuls," but nobody can know for sure in advance. Bringing them into the pool under liberal admission criteria can't be helped if we want to increase the chances of uncovering hidden talent. In other words, the imperfections in our measures force us to make a choice between overincluding the non-gifted and overexcluding the gifted, and it is safer to err on the side of overinclusion.[13]

The other implication of the imprecision in identifying giftedness is that we are very likely to be wasting our time and money by becoming overly formalized in identification procedures. For the little predictive power that they possess, administering intelligence tests to large numbers of children is a wasteful undertaking. In addition to their imprecision, intelligence tests don't measure the interests and motivations that are most crucial to giftedness.

In order to achieve a comprehensive assessment of children, it is more valuable to provide informal activities through which children have the opportunity to demonstrate their interests as well as abilities. Spatial-mechanical activities can be used in the classroom so that a teacher has the opportunity to observe behaviors related to the five components of accomplishment, i.e. a strong interest, appropriate abilities, appropriate imagination, sustained activity, and independence of thought.

Teachers should feel free to create their own activities, but I can mention a few possibilities as examples:

1. If there are mechanical type construction sets of various kinds in the classroom for students to use in their free time, a teacher can observe which students use these materials most, the degree of complexity they achieve in their designs, and the uniqueness of the designs. This is most important for early elementary children and could include block building, Tinker toys,® erector sets, and Lego sets.

2. When a teacher uses the spatial concept training programs developed by Anita Harnadek and by Howard and Sandra Black, this gives many opportunities to observe those

children who catch on quickly and have a high motivation level in the activities.[14] Barbara Ryan, a teacher of gifted children in the Stamford, Connecticut public schools, has found the greatest differences between children emerge when, after using the Harnadek and Black materials, children are asked to create their own figural analogies and spatial transformation activities.

3. In her *Challenge Box* program, Catherine Valentino describes several different activities that would be useful for assessing the mechanical interests and imagination of students.[15] In one activity, students are asked to explain, "What happens when you put 30 cents into a Coke® machine? How does the Coke machine know you didn't put in 20 cents?" (or 40 cents or 10 cents). In another activity students are shown a pop-up book for children and are asked to design one of their own. In a third activity students are asked to invent a method for measuring an hour of time with water.

4. E. Paul Torrance has described creative activities that involve spatial-mechanical interest.[16] In one activity, students are asked to explain the workings of an unfamiliar educational toy. In another activity, they are asked to redesign toys. The emphasis in these activities is on unique ideas, but a teacher could also look for complexity of structural thinking that would be an indication of spatial ability and interest.

5. Any graphic arts activities or science activities that require the manipulation of materials gives a teacher opportunities to see which students have a particularly good sense of how to relate materials to each other so that they hang together and make sense.

These informal activities might not give a teacher a precise measure that compares the ability of a child with the general population. They do give a teacher opportunities to observe interest and the tendency in some children to stay with a spatial-mechanical problem for an extended period of time. These motivational observations are probably more important than any precise test scores.

A teacher should be most interested in those students who have not performed particularly well in more formal academic subjects.

These are the children who could be particularly helped by recognition of their spatial-mechanical abilities, interests, and imaginations.

IF FORMAL ASSESSMENTS ARE NECESSARY
— FOR ELEMENTARY STUDENTS

Many states and many school systems require that some standardized documentation be available before a student can be served in a program for gifted children. Sometimes an IQ score at a certain level is required, such as an IQ of 130 or above. In other places, it is necessary to demonstrate that a student is among the top 2, 3, 4, or 5 percent of the local school population in ability. When these requirements exist, it is necessary to employ some standardized testing procedures.

If gifted spatial children are going to be allowed to enter programs through such procedures, it is important that one testing issue be dealt with. Spatial children will rarely achieve a comprehensive IQ score that meets the criterion of most localities. In addition to their strengths, most spatial children have weakness in some areas of ability, especially those related to formal language. This being the case, their average comprehensive IQ scores will rarely meet regulation standards. If these children are to enter programs for the gifted, it is essential that the criteria be adjusted to accept children with specific areas of strength. A spatial IQ of 130 must be considered an appropriate indicator of potential giftedness. It is therefore essential that a multifactor IQ test battery be employed so that separate components of ability can be observed.

Another issue that must be dealt with is the fact that a large portion of spatial children will still not meet the criteria for being considered "officially" gifted. Even though spatial ability may be the primary strength of this larger group of children, they won't necessarily have spatial IQ scores in the top 2 percent or 5 percent of the population. One could, of course, insist that research fails to support the restrictive criteria written into the laws and that the potential for giftedness should be considered a more wide-open probability game as suggested by Abraham Tannenbaum.[17] From a more practical point of view, however, it is probably better to accept the unfortunate fact that the restrictive laws are likely to be in place for some time to come. It is better to simply make arrangements to see that spatial children are appropriately served whether or not they can officially participate in programs for the gifted.

In the selection of gifted students, several comprehensive IQ assessment systems are available. There is no question, however, that the Wechsler Intelligence Scales for Children (WISC-R) is the most widely used system and the one for which most research information is available. The WISC-R is, therefore, recommended for assessing skill patterns among elementary school children.

Lucile Beckman has produced strong evidence that the WISC-R can be of value in identifying spatial children.[18] Beckman asked mathematics teachers to divide children into two groups on whether the children learned better by using manipulative materials to represent mathematics concepts or learned better from verbal explanations. In addition, Beckman obtained scores from the block design subtest of the WISC-R. The block design subtest turned out to be a very accurate indicator of whether a child learned better through manipulative materials or through verbal explanation. This can be seen in Table 7-I.

Table 7-I

Numbers of Students in Beckman's Research Classified by Whether They Learned Best Through Manipulative Materials and by Whether They Achieved a High Score on Block Design

Block Design Score Level	Learned Best Using Manipulative Materials	Learned Best from Verbal Explanations
Block design score of 16 or over	32	8
Block design score under 16	2	16

Considering that Beckman used only one subtest and that there was no comparison of spatial ability to verbal ability, these results are quite impressive. They give confidence in the use of the WISC-R for identifying spatial children. It would be recommended, however, that the full WISC-R battery be employed so that reliability of testing can be assured and so that a comparison between different aspects of ability can be made.

There have been many studies of patterns in WISC-R scores. McLeod's review of several studies was mentioned in Chapter 3.[19] McLeod was interested in the WISC-R patterns for dyslexic children. Although only a small portion of spatial children would be considered dyslexic in a formal sense, the skill patterns of the two groups tend to be associated. McLeod found there was rather high consistency in the skill patterns derived from the eight studies reviewed.

Tests on which Dyslexic Children Performed Well	*Tests on which Dyslexic Children Performed Poorly*
Block design	Digit span
Picture arrangement	Information
Comprehension	Arithmetic
Picture completion	Coding
Similarities	
Object assembly	

Alexander Bannatyne has devised his own way of grouping WISC-R subtests based on his work with learning-disabled children and on his factor-analytic studies.[20]

Spatial	*Verbal Conceptualization*	*Acquired Knowledge*	*Sequencing*
Picture completion	Similarities	Information	Arithmetic
Block design	Vocabulary	Arithmetic	Digit span
Object assembly	Comprehension	Vocabulary	Coding

In the Bannatyne classification, the magnitude of test scores for spatial children will tend to go in order from left to right with spatial tests scores being highest and sequencing test scores being lowest.

In using this information from McLeod and Bannatyne, it needs to be remembered that all spatial children are not learning-disabled, and all learning-disabled children are not spatial children. A similarity in test score patterns for spatial children and a portion of learning-disabled children is all that is implied here. Clements and Peters have found that the skill patterns of the wider group of learning-disabled children follow three different patterns.[21] Only one of these three corresponds to the pattern for spatial children.

Factor-analytic study of WISC-R test scores from the wider population of children arrives at similar distinctions. Alan Kaufman has perhaps conducted the most comprehensive set of these studies.[22] After factor-analyzing test scores for several age groups, Kaufman concluded that the more satisfactory way to group subtests is as follows:

Perceptual Organization	*Verbal Comprehension*	*Freedom from Distractibility*
Picture completion	Information	Arithmetic
Picture arrangement	Similarities	Digit span
Block design	Vocabulary	Coding
Object Assembly	Comprehension	
Mazes		

Working from these various sources of information, I would arrive at the following grouping of WISC-R subtests as being most relevant to identifying spatial children:

Spatial Gestalt	*Gestalt Sequencing*	*Verbal Comprehension*	*Detailed Memory and Sequencing*
Block design	Picture arrangement	Similarities	Information
Picture completion	Mazes	Vocabulary	Digit span
Object assembly		Comprehension	Coding
			Arithmetic

When identifying spatial children, one should first look for a distinct superiority in *spatial gestalt* subtest scores over *detailed memory and sequencing* scores. On the WISC-R subtest the national normed score mean is 10 and the standard deviation is 3. The scores for the *spatial gestalt* subtest should tend to be 3 or more points above the *detailed memory and sequencing* subtests in order to conclude that there is a distinct superiority. For spatial children the *gestalt sequencing* tests will tend to be second in order of magnitude and the *verbal comprehension* scores will be third.

In looking for this kind of pattern, it should be remembered that the reliability in individual subtest scores is not very great. This means that one or two individual subtest scores can deviate from the general pattern without indicating that the general pattern is not present. One should never expect to find a completely consistent pattern for an individual child.

Some spatial children may show distinct indications of giftedness in spatial abilities. In this case, their spatial gestalt scores will tend to

be above 13. Other spatial children will be more average in spatial
ability. Their scores will tend to range from 9 to 13. The first group
might qualify for gifted education programs when criteria for participation are rigidly defined. The second group might not qualify
for a gifted education program. It must be remembered, however,
that the strengths of this second group are in spatial gestalt abilities.
This will have important implications for their most efficient learning mode. The research of Lucile Beckman has indicated that these
children learn best through spatial representation of concepts.

IF FORMAL ASSESSMENTS ARE NECESSARY
— FOR HIGH SCHOOL STUDENTS

Just as the WISC-R is the most widely used test for elementary
school students, the Differential Aptitude Tests (DAT) is the most
widely used battery for high school students. The 1972 revision of
this battery has eight subtests; these allow for a reliable indication of
varying skill patterns.

Verbal reasoning
Numerical ability
Abstract reasoning
Clerical speed and accuracy
Mechanical reasoning
Space relations
Spelling
Language usage

The DAT has the advantage of being group-administered and
group-scored. It is economical to test all children at a given grade
level.

The space relations subtest is a good measure of spatial ability.
The mechanical reasoning subtest is closely related to spatial ability,
but does rely much more on the experience of a student. The
subtests least related to spatial ability are language usage, clerical
speed and accuracy, verbal reasoning, and spelling. The remaining
two subtests, abstract reasoning and numerical ability, relate to both
spatial ability and verbal ability and therefore cannot be placed
distinctly in either group. Factor-analytic study of the DAT suggests
that, when looking for spatial children, the following group of tests

should be used[23].

Spatial	*General*	
Mechanical	*Intellectual*	*Verbal Detailed*
Space relations	Numerical ability	Language usage
Mechanical reasoning	Abstract reasoning	Clerical speed and accuracy
		Verbal reasoning
		Spelling

In the score patterns for spatial children, the spatial-mechanical test scores will tend to be distinctly superior to the verbal-detailed test scores. The general intellectual tests will tend to fall somewhere between, sometimes relating more to the spatial-mechanical tests and other times more to the verbal-detailed tests. Again, it should be remembered that individual subtest scores have a low level of reliability and the deviation of one or two individual scores from the general pattern does not invalidate the pattern.

A TEACHER CHECKLIST

Over the past several years, attempts have been made to create personality checklists based on cerebral asymmetry research. These checklists can be used to relate behavioral characteristics to spatial and verbal ability differences. The research on these checklists has not reached the point where it is possible to say that they provide reliable guides to school programming. Nevertheless, an observational checklist can provide confirmatory indications that the result obtained from activities and testing match general behavioral characteristics.

One very interesting checklist has been created by Fadely and Hosler. The checklist consists of 100 items and is intended to be filled out by teachers, when a teacher has the time to deal with an 100 item checklist. The checklist can be used as it appears in the Fadely and Hosler book. In many school situations such an involved checklist would be difficult to use. I have, therefore, restructured the Fadely and Hosler checklist to create a seven-item version that is much easier to use. In this seven-item version, each item was created by merging several of the Fadely and Hosler items.

On the restructured checklist, teachers are asked to assess the extent to which a child goes in one direction or another on characteristics that are often in opposition to each other. The characteristics on the right side of each item are associated with right hemisphere thinking as understood by Fadely and Hosler.[24]

CEREBRAL DOMINANCE OBSERVATION GUIDE*

The descriptions on the left side and on the right side of each item below give groups of characteristics that often go together in a child. Sometimes a child can distinctly be described by the characteristics on the left side of an item or by those on the right side. Other children are rather well balanced between the two descriptions. Please indicate the extent to which a child goes in one direction or the other by circling the appropriate position.

I.

Has good vocabulary, speaks grammatically, good at answering questions, uses good order in expression of thoughts, asks for verbal information.

VERBALLY EXPRESSIVE

Enjoys physical activity and making things, relates to others in physical ways, talks with gestures, restless in verbally structured situations.

MOTORICALLY EXPRESSIVE

Mostly   Somewhat   Balanced   Somewhat   Mostly

II.

Is conventionally objective and moral, deliberately sets goals in conventional ways, accepts reasons for social rules.

LOGICAL

Is sensitive, moody, introspective, dreamy, senses earthy side of problems, responds to music and other sensory mood-setting stimuli.

INTUITIVE

Mostly   Somewhat   Balanced   Somewhat   Mostly

III.

Remembers and follows directions, is well organized, has orderly, sequential thought patterns, anticipates and cares about consequences of behavior.

Appreciates complexities in a global way without attention to details, tries to express larger meanings with few words, sensitive to the physical wholeness of

*Modified from J.L. Fadely and V.N. Hosler, *Understanding the Alpha Child at Home and School.* Springfield, Ill.: Charles C Thomas, Publisher, 1979.

people, objects, and things, but
misses details and forgets names.

SEQUENTIAL THINKING			WHOLISTIC THINKING	
Mostly	Somewhat	Balanced	Somewhat	Mostly

IV.

Has an orderly sense of days, weeks, months, and time of day, adheres to schedules and organizes time in a systematic way.

Has a strong visual memory for events but little memory for dates or time, good sense of the surrounding world and movement in it, enjoys open space and lack of crowding.

TIME ORIENTATION			SPATIAL ORIENTATION	
Mostly	Somewhat	Balanced	Somewhat	Mostly

V.

Stresses appropriate behavior and rules of right or wrong, expresses remorse for misbehavior, wants social acceptance, has socially acceptable goals.

Develops values according to situation not convention, needs immediate gratification, feels a oneness with everything, has shifting friendships depending on mood.

SOCIALIZED VALUES			NATURALISTIC VALUES	
Mostly	Somewhat	Balanced	Somewhat	Mostly

VI.

Is assertive with others, wants to compete, pushes cooperative activity, uses conventional rules to control others, wants to achieve.

Accepts but isn't strongly committed to others, dislikes aggressiveness, compromises, changes goals when blocked, resists control by others when trapped.

ASSERTIVE				ACCEPTING
Mostly	Somewhat	Balanced	Somewhat	Mostly

VII.

Applies known values to problems, good at understanding familiar problems, classifies information in usual ways, understands social behavior.

Is imaginative, enjoys fantasy, has unusual ideas, elaborates on thoughts outside of the usual, visualizes new things, is not socially astute.

STRUCTURED THOUGHT			CREATIVE THOUGHT	
Mostly	Somewhat	Balanced	Somewhat	Mostly

If a child can be most appropriately described by the descriptive statements on the right side of the Fadely-Hosler observation guide (revised), and if this corresponds to a specialized strength and motivation in spatial-mechanical activities, teachers and parents can be quite certain they have identified a spatial child. There are, however, good reasons why the two might not correspond for a given child. In the first place, we have very limited knowledge of the relationships between abilities and the personality patterns described by Fadely and Hosler. Also, children are strongly influenced by the social environment, and sometimes their personalities are shaped away from their most natural inclinations.

Many spatial children come under considerable pressure to be somewhat different from the way they are internally inclined. In some cases this may be necessary in order to facilitate social adjustment. In other cases, the pressures may go far beyond anything that can be logically justified, and the pressures may derive more from the compulsive sensitivities of adults than from the legitimate need for social order.

Although the Fadely and Hosler checklist is valuable for understanding variations in the personalities of children, when the spatial ability strengths of a child do not correspond to right-minded characteristics on the checklist, the ability strengths are definitely more central to the identification of spatial children. Perhaps the greatest value of the checklist is that it sensitizes teachers and parents to varying personality characteristics in children.

A SELF-DESCRIPTIVE CHECKLIST
FOR OLDER CHILDREN

Another checklist based on cerebral asymmetry research has been created by Torrance, Riegel, and Reynolds.[25] As opposed to the Fadely and Hosler checklist, the Torrance, Riegel, and Reynolds checklist is a self-descriptive one intended to be filled out by the child. Since children younger than age ten don't tend to have the introspectiveness required to fill out such a questionnaire, it is recommended that it be used only with older children. The Torrance, Riegel, and Reynolds checklist seems a little complex in its original form for convenient use. I have therefore created a slightly simplified revision of the checklist. The answers on the right side of each item are associated with right hemisphere thinking.

DIXON LEARNING AND
THINKING PREFERENCE INVENTORY*

Some people do one thing better and some do other things better. In order for us to be good teachers, we need to know what kinds of things you do best.

Below are twenty-one questions. For each question, choose between the two answers. It may be difficult deciding which answer to choose because people can often do many things well.

Even if it is difficult, make the best choice. For each question circle the one answer that is most like you.

1. Do you remember names better or faces better?
   Names   Faces

2. Do you understand how to do something better if someone explains it to you, or if someone demonstrates how it is done?
   Explains   Demonstrates

3. Do you feel comfortable telling people right away how you feel about things, or does it take a special effort?
   Feel Comfortable   Special Effort

4. Do you like multiple choice tests better, or do you like tests where you have to write the answer?
   Write Answer   Multiple Choice

5. Do you like classes in which you can be active and do things, or classes in which you listen to others?
   Listen   Active

6. Are you more likely to decide things on the basis of what others tell you about it, or on the basis of personal experiences and hunches about it?
   What Others Tell Me   Personal Experience

7. Do you enjoy playing around at finding answers to problems, or do you want to know one right away?
   One Right Way   Playing Around

8. Are you better at thinking of ideas if you are alone to concentrate, or do you think things through better when you are with

---

*Modified from Torrance, E. Paul, Riegel, Theodore, and Reynolds, Cecil R. In Torrance, E.P., *Your Style of Learning and Thinking*. Athens, Georgia,.

groups of other people?
With Other People   Alone to Concentrate

9. Are you usually able to use what things are available to get a job done, or do you prefer to use the right materials that were intended for the job?
Right Materials   Things Available

10. Do you tend to have more new and different ideas than other people, or not so many?
Not So Many   More New Ideas

11. Do you think best when you are sitting upright, or do you think better when you are lying down or walking?
Sitting Upright   Lying Down or Walking

12. Do you like to solve problems that are straightforward, or ones that are complicated?
Straightforward   Complicated

13. Do you prefer to learn about things that are known for sure, or do you enjoy learning about new and different ideas which are not so certain?
Known for Sure   New Uncertain Ideas

14. Do you like to solve problems by picturing in your mind the things involved in the problems, or would you rather talk about the things involved in the problem?
Talking   Picturing

15. When you are trying to help someone understand how to do something, do you do better by talking to them about it, or by showing them through action how to do it?
Talking   Showing

16. Do you depend more on names and words for remembering things, or do you depend more on pictures in your mind?
Names and Words   Pictures In My Mind

17. Do you like trying to understand something that other people have done, or would you rather try completing something of your own?
Understanding What Others   Completing Something of
Have Done   My Own

18. Which do you enjoy more, talking and writing or drawing and making things?
Talking and Writing   Drawing and Making
                             Things

19. When you are in a strange place, do you tend to get lost easily or do you tend to find your way around easily?
    Get Lost Easily   Find Way Easily

20. When you are studying a subject, do you like to learn lots of facts, or do you like to concentrate on a few important facts which help you get the whole picture of what the subject is about?
    Lots of Facts   Important Facts for Whole Picture

21. Do you tend to accept and appreciate what you hear and read, or do you tend more to search, question and think on your own?
    Accept What I Hear and Read   Think On My Own

Neither the *Cerebral Dominance Observation Guide* or the *Dixon Learning and Thinking Preference Inventory* should be used as an exclusive method for identifying spatial children. Both have been created on the basis of an assortment of research on cerebral asymmetry. Their relationship to spatial ability is indirect. The checklists should be used only as a backup for other information collected on a child and as a means of achieving a fuller understanding of the child's cognitive style.

GENERAL CONCLUSIONS ON IDENTIFICATION

Under ideal circumstances, identification of spatial children should be treated as a flexible, open process involving natural activities and natural observations on the child. In almost any school subject it is possible to include spatial-mechanical activities. For example, even in a history or social studies class, it is possible to have some activities that involve construction of models representing the way of life of people at different time periods and different locations. It is then possible to discover children who are particularly good and particularly creative at the spatial-mechanical aspects of these activities.

It is perhaps most important to make observations on the motivational levels of students during these activities. When one notices a child who is usually not very motivated for most school work getting highly involved in spatial-mechanical activities, this child is almost certainly a spatial child in some sense. This type of child, perhaps more than any others, needs attending to with understanding of his spatial-mechanical preference in approaching the world. Chapters 8 through 11 present a variety of curricular ideas that are helpful in maximizing the school performance of this type of child.

REFERENCES

1. Renzulli, J.S., Reis, S.M., and Smith, L.H. *The Revolving Door Identification Model.* Mansfield, Conn.: Creative Learning Press, 1981; Tannenbaum, A.J., and Baldwin, L.J. *Giftedness and Learning Disability: A Paradoxical Combination.* Unpublished manuscript, Columbia University, 1982.
2. Polak, F.L. *The Images of the Future.* New York: Elsevier, 1973; Singer, B.D. The future focused role image. In Toffler, A. *Learning for Tomorrow.* New York: Vintage, 1974; Torrance, E.P. Creativity and futurism in education. *Education, 100*:298-311, 1980.
3. Torrance, E.P. *Some Implications of Creativity Research for Gifted Education.* Paper presented at the Second Conference on Creativity in Gifted Education. Memphis, Tenn., March 21, 1981.
4. Goleman, D. The new competency tests. *Psychology Today, 15*:35-46, 1981.
5. Renzulli, *op. cit.,* p. 28.
6. Reitan, R.M., and Davison, L.A. *Clinical Neuropsychology: Current Status and Applications.* New York: John Wiley, 1974, pp. 20-21.
7. Prentky, R.A. *Creativity and Psychopathology.* New York: Praeger Publishers, 1980, p. 129.
8. Renzulli, *op. cit.,* pp. 24-26.
9. Roe, A. *The Making of a Scientist.* New York: Dodd, Mead, 1952.
10. Stone, I. *The Origin.* New York: New American Library, 1981, p. 8.
11. *Ibid.,* p. 36.
12. Renzulli, *op. cit.,* p. 26.
13. Tannenbaum and Baldwin, *op. cit.* p. 1.
14. Harnadek, A. *Spatial Perception.* Pacific Grove, Calif.: Midwest Publications, 1979; Black, H., and Black, S. *Figural Analogies.* Pacific Grove, Calif.: Midwest Publications, 1981.
15. Valentino, C. *Challenge Boxes.* West Kingston, R.I.
16. Torrance, E.P. Education and creativity. In Rothenberg, A. and Hausman, C.R. *The Creativity Question.* Durham, N.C.: Duke University Press, 1976, pp. 217-227.
17. Tannenbaum and Baldwin, *op. cit.,* p. 1.
18. Beckman, L. Use of the block design sub-test of the WISC as an instrument for identifying children who prefer a non-verbal (spatial) approach to learning. In Gallagher, J. *Gifted Children: Reaching Their Potential.* Jerusalem, Israel: Kollek and Son, 1979, pp. 211-222.
19. McLeod, J. A comparison of WISC sub-test scores of pre-adolescent successful and unsuccessful readers. *Australian Journal of Psychology, 17*:220-228, 1965.

20. Bannatyne, A. Diagnosis: a note on recategorization of the WISC scaled scores. *Journal of Learning Disabilities, 7*:272-274, 1974.

21. Clements, S., and Peters, J. Minimal brain dysfunction in the school age child. In Frierson, E., and Barbe, W. *Educating Children with Learning Disabilities*. New York: Appleton Century Crofts, 1967.

22. Kaufman, A. Factor analysis of the WISC-R at eleven age levels between six and one half and sixteen and one half years. *Journal of Consulting and Clinical Psychology, 43*:135-147, 1975.

23. Cooper, M. Factor analysis of measures of aptitude, intelligence, personality, and performance in high school subjects. *Journal of Experimental Education, 42*:7-10, 1974.

24. Fadely, J.L., and Hosler, V.N. *Understanding the Alpha Child at Home and School*. Springfield, Ill.: Charles C Thomas, Publisher, 1979, pp. 150-154.

25. Torrance, E.P. *Your Style of Learning and Thinking*. Georgia Studies of Creative Behavior, 185 Riverhill Drive, Athens, Georgia 30601.

Chapter 8

ENCOURAGING STRENGTHS

SPATIALLY BASED ACTIVITIES

PERHAPS more important than any other element in the education of a spatial child is the opportunity to be involved in activities that are of interest to the child and activities at which the
child is very competent. This allows the child to develop those skills
that are most likely to form the foundation for adult accomplishment. It also gives the child opportunities to feel comfortable about
his abilities. Building self-regard in a child who has been taught
from an early age to have doubts about his abilities can be the key to
successful teaching.

When Sir Isaac Newton, after an inappropriate overdose of
classical languages as a child, was finally able to focus on the scientific ideas that he loved, this turned his academic performance
around from failure to success and became the basis for the flowering
of his genius. Pablo Picasso's father accepted the fact that his son
would never be a scholar and allowed his son to study art full-time.
This laid the foundation for the most financially successful artistic
career in history. The fact that Albert Einstein somehow managed to
be accepted as a student at the Swiss Federal Polytechnic School
after his prior failures in school salvaged a life headed toward
miserable impotence. To Auguste Rodin's sister, who supported his
desire to study art in spite of lack of confidence by his parents that he
was capable of doing anything very well, we are in debt for some of
the greatest sculpture of all time.

We should learn from these lessons. There is no established
means by which children can be helped to discover their strengths.
There are several approaches that are being used and that seem from
experience to work for the children involved. The first element in
any effort to encourage spatial children should be the availability of a
good graphic arts program and a good natural science program.
Although spatial children do not always achieve in the graphic arts
and sciences, history and experience indicate that these are the most

176

likely areas of exceptional achievement. A graphic arts program should allow for the imaginative use of materials. A physical science program should emphasize learning through experimentation rather than through memorizing terms, principles, and formulas.

If a woodworking or craft studio is available, spatial children will often enjoy this kind of activity. At the Whitby School in Greenwich, Connecticut, children are allowed to choose their own activities for about half of the school day. Among the choices is a woodworking shop. The teachers at the school have found that learning-disabled students are more likely than other students to choose woodworking as an activity and that many of these children are particularly creative at their artistic and construction projects.

It is also useful to have children study the nature of spatial relationships in a formal way. Materials for this purpose have been created by Anita Harnadek, Sandra Black, and Howard Black.[1] The skills taught in the Harnadek and Black materials are essentially identical to skills involved in the commonly used spatial tests. The principal difference between these materials and tests is that some spatial vocabulary is taught with the activities, and the activities are sequenced to go from very simple concepts and manipulations to rather challenging ones.

Spatial concepts should definitely be emphasized in a mathematics program. Lucile Beckman has demonstrated in her research that children whose primary strengths are in spatial abilities are helped by a mathematics program based on spatial, manipulative materials and concepts.[2] Many good mathematics programs of this type have been developed. Mary Laycock and Gene Watson of the Nueva Day School and Learning Center in Hillsborough, California, have developed an exceptional program.[3] The Nuffield Mathematics series on shape and size has a strong base in spatial concepts.[4] Using spatial concepts, the Nuffield series takes children all the way from simple counting to the geometry of polyhedra. In selecting these types of materials, it is important to distinguish between those programs that stress only the manipulative nature of the materials and those that develop the understanding of spatial relationships. Manipulative materials can be useful in teaching computational concepts, but an understanding of spatial structure is much more involved than that. The grasp of spatial gestalt structure is the area in which spatial children can be most distinguished, and the effort to stress a child's strengths must move to that level if it is to be most productive.

CREATIVE DEVELOPMENT

The above ideas on the development of spatial abilities are rather obvious, and related materials are available through a variety of sources. There is another area of strength that is more subtle and that merits more consideration. Evidence was presented in Chapter 6 for the conclusion that spatial children have an inclination toward unusual creative production. In making this assertion, it is important to distinguish between different kinds of creativity. Spatial children are more likely to be adept at creativity involving gestalt transformations than at creativity that stresses ideational fluency. The relationship between spatial ability and creativity is not well understood, but those who work with spatial children generally agree that an inclination toward unique ideas is often present.[5]

There is considerable available knowledge on the nature and needs of creative children, and we should take heed of these ideas in our work with spatial children. The research of Getzels and Jackson has established a somewhat classic view of the creative child, and it is worth taking note of their conclusions. In order to clarify the characteristics of creatively productive children as distinguished from children who are intelligent in more conventional ways, Getzels and Jackson selected two groups of children. In one group, the children had achieved distinctly high scores on tests of creativity but not such high scores on a test of intellectual ability. In the second group, the children had achieved high scores on an IQ test, but not such high scores on tests of creativity. The contrasts in the personality characteristics of the two groups were sharp, and have provided a guideline for those who work with highly creative children.

> It seems to us that the essence of the performance of our creative adolescents lay in their ability to produce new forms, to risk conjoining elements that are customarily thought of as independent and dissimilar, to "go off in new directions." The creative adolescent seemed to possess the ability to free himself from the usual, to "diverge" from the customary. He seemed to enjoy the risk and uncertainty of the unknown. In contrast, the high I.Q. adolescent seemed to possess to a high degree the ability and the need to focus on the usual, to be channeled and controlled in the direction of the right answer — the customary. He appeared to shy away

from the risk and the uncertainty of the unknown and to seek out the safe-
ty and security of the known. Furthermore, and most important, these
differences do not seem to be restricted to the cognitive functioning of
these two groups. The data with respect to both intellectually oriented and
socially oriented behavior are of a piece. . . . The high I.Q.'s tend to converge upon stereotyped meanings, to perceive personal success by conventional standards, to move toward the model provided by teachers, to seek
out careers that conform to what is expected of them. The high creatives
tend to diverge from stereotyped meanings, to produce original fantasies,
to perceive personal success by unconventional standards, to seek out
careers that do not conform to what is expected of them.[6]

Creative children can suffer considerably when their special inclinations are not respected. Their principal need is for opportunities
to develop that native talent. For a general source of information on
researched approaches to creative development, I can recommend
Developing Creativity in the Gifted and Talented by Carolyn Callahan.[7] In
addition, I can briefly review six aspects of creative process that
should be kept in mind when working toward creative development.
These six aspects are environmental awareness, problem sensitivity,
deeper levels of internal awareness, recognizing patterns and connections, risk taking, and organizing social networks to support
divergent thought processes.

One would have difficulty naming any creative production that
didn't in some way involve sensitivity to a phenomenon that most
other people were either not seeing at all or overlooking as being of
no significance. This is so much the case that William James concluded that "genius in truth means little more than the faculty of
perceiving in an unhabitual way."[8] To some extent, this capacity is
intrinsic to the creative child, and all we need to do as teachers is
recognize when it is happening so we may encourage expression of
insights by the child. On the other hand, it is always helpful to carry
on classroom activities that allow creative children to use this ability
and that give them the opportunity to experience reinforcement for
their insights. Good example activities are given in Linda Allison's
book, *Blood And Guts: A Working Guide To Your Own Little Insides*.[9]

Often associated with this special sense of environmental
awareness are insights into problems that most people do not see.
This involves discovery of a deficiency in conventional wisdom that
other people are refusing to deal with. For example, Einstein was led
to develop his special theory of relativity because he was willing

to focus on a piece of information that didn't conform to existing assumptions about the working of the universe. Most other scientists who knew of it were ready to either ignore the information or to suggest that it was wrong. After gaining fame for his work, Einstein went so far as to suggest that "the formulation of a problem is often more essential than its solution, which may be merely a matter of mathematical or experimental skill. To raise new questions, new problems, to regard old problems from a new angle, requires creative imagination and marks real advance in science."[10] An interesting exploration of this idea has been provided by Getzels and Csikszentmihalyi in their study of art students.[11] A creative development program that starts with problem sensitivity as its core element has been provided by Sidney Parnes at the Creative Education Foundation.[12]

It has long been known that many creative insights derive from deep levels of human consciousness. Flashes of insight sometimes come in a quiet moment when one is resting or walking or on vacation — when the more surface levels of consciousness are not actively engaged. Sometimes creative products are the result of dreams or come in a half-awake state. So prominent and common are the descriptions of these experiences in the biographical literature that when Wallas made his landmark effort to set out the stages of the creative process in 1926, two of his four stages had to do with this experience. One of these he called incubation and the other illumination. About incubation he said —

> . . . that a series of unconscious and involuntary (or foreconscious and forevoluntary) mental events may take place during that period . . . in the case of the more difficult forms of creative thought, the making, for instance, of a scientific discovery, or the writing of a poem or play or the formulation of an important political decision, it is desirable not only that there should be an interval free from conscious thought on the particular problem concerned, but also that the interval should be so spent that nothing should interfere with the free working of the unconscious or partially conscious process of the mind.[13]

The next stage, illumination, is that sudden point at which one realizes the product of the relatively unconscious mental work that has been taking place.

> Helmholtz and Poincare both speak of the appearance of a new idea as instantaneous and unexpected. If we so define the illumination stage as to restrict it to this instantaneous "flash," it is obvious that we cannot

influence it by a direct effort of will; because we can only bring our will to bear upon psychological events which last for an appreciable time. On the other hand, the final "flash," or "click," is the culmination of a successful train of association, which may have lasted for an appreciable time, and which has probably been preceded by a series of tentative and unsuccessful trains . . . both the unsuccessful trains of association, which might have led to the "flash" of success, and the final and successful train are normally either unconscious, or take place (with "risings" and "fallings" of consciousness as success seems to appoach or retire), in that periphery or "fringe" of consciousness which surrounds our "focal" consciousness as the sun's "corona" surrounds the disk of full luminosity.[14]

There is considerable evidence that suggests that our inner minds are continually at work in a way we are hardly aware of and that these inner workings are not well known to us until we limit the intake of external stimulation. Although the inner workings of our minds are always somewhat available to us, it is not until we stop to rest or are doing something to quiet the outer workings that we become aware of the deeper levels of consciousness.[15] There is also evidence that our inner minds use a special language, a metaphoric coding and patterning, of which we are most aware from our dreaming.[16] The creative work of our inner minds takes place in this little understood metaphoric code. The Freudians started us on the road to unraveling this code, but then proceeded to lead everyone astray by oversexualizing their interpretations. Psychologists are just beginning to get back on the track of understanding the inner mind as a general problem solver, perhaps something like a special computer that operates with its own natural language and logical connections. Before it can operate, information must be translated into its language, and before we can benefit from its knowledge, its messages must be translated back into our outer language and categories of working consciousness. Such translation is more likely to take place at special moments of quiet and relaxation when we are not overwhelmed by incoming information. The testimony for this position is considerable; attested to by such mental giants as the philosopher-mathematician Descartes, the physicist Helmholtz, and the mathematician Poincare. Newton's creativity when forced by a plague to be away from the university, Darwin's creativity when in bed due to chronic illness, and Einstein's evident benefits from lying for hours in his sailboat would also support this claim.

The value of internal awareness has not been adequately explored in relation to the school context. Some sources of ideas can be found in *The Inner World Of Daydreaming* by Jerome Singer and *Seeing With The Mind's Eye* by Mike and Nancy Samuels.[17]

Perhaps the most challenging aspects of creative process is the recognition of patterns and connections. If the right hemisphere does play a special role in creativity, it is probably in this area: seeing the gestalt, the holistic patterning of things. It is very difficult to generalize about this because the nature of patterning and connecting is always specific to a given area of endeavor. It is dependent on a broad factual knowledge of a given subject. This relates to the fact that creative people are often collectors of information and things; collectors of things about which they have only a vague inkling of future use. Charles Darwin was a collector of natural phenomena from a young age. Albert Einstein's years of experience as a patent clerk in the Swiss Patent Office contributed considerably to his source of creatively suggestive information. Charles Townes, the chief developer of the laser, has been noted throughout his life as a collector of things. As a boy, he was stamp collector, a butterfly collector, and a collector of bottlecaps. As a college student, he ran the small museum at his college. As an adult he was a collector of facts about the electromagnetic spectrum. His broad knowledge of how microwaves interact with molecules led to his success as an inventor.[18] The music composer, John Gage, got started in his most creative work after a friend convinced him that a knowledge of sounds in general could be a source of insight — that everything in the world, even silence, has its own sound.

The key element in patterning and connecting, however, is not simply possessing the facts. It is what is done with the facts. The information must be sorted and sifted so that underlying patterns begin to appear. Buckminister Fuller described this aspect of his thinking: "I am a swimmer and a dismisser of irrelevancies. Everything we need to work with is around us, although most of it is initially confusing. To find order in what we experience we must first inventory the total experience, then temporarily set aside all irrelevancies. I do not invent my thoughts. I merely separate out some local patterns from a confusing whole."[19]

There is no general source of ideas about teaching these patterning and connecting processes. Perhaps, it is the inner core of creativity and least understood. There are, however, three special ways of making connections that have been studied and that are somewhat understood. These are metaphoric thinking, analogical thinking, and paradoxical thinking. Metaphors and analogies are very similar. They rest on the recognition that one situation has characteristics and relationships that are similar to some other situation not ordinarily associated with the first. Knowledge of how things work in the first situation can then be suggestive of how things could work in the second. A popular example of this is Alexander Bell's analogy between the workings of the ear and the workings of his telephone receiver. A suggested way to approach this kind of thinking is called morphological analysis. After a problem area has been decided on, the ingredients, characteristics, and relationships are then listed. These components are then described in the most general way possible (e.g. an eardrum is something that vibrates when struck by sound waves). One can then think of other situations that share the generalizations. (What other things vibrate when struck by sound waves?) Insights very often evolve out of this kind of thought process.

Paradox leads to insights in a somewhat different way. A paradox is a situation where two things appear to be true, and at the same time are contradictory to each other. "Religion teaches men to be good, conscientious beings. Yet religion throughout history has been the source of some of the most brutal conflicts." Discovery of the source of contradictions leads to deeper levels of understanding and creativity. Two sources of ideas on teaching for the discovery of patterns and connections would be *The Art of the Possible* by W.J.J. Gordon and Tony Poze and *Classroom Ideas for Encouraging Thinking and Feeling* by Frank Williams.[20]

In the process of creative production, having new and different ideas is not sufficient to assure that the ideas become useful. Many people generate creative ideas that are never used. There is a certain riskiness about promoting new ideas. In the extensive studies of creative people by Frank Barron and Donald MacKinnon, one clearly consistent aspect of the creative personality was the willingness to take risks.[21] In pursuing their imaginative ideas, creative people have little concern for how they are perceived by others. Their disregard for social convention is very much like that of mentally deviant people. This risky relationship to social convention may seem romantic when it is spoken of in sterilized clinical terms, but when we are talking of the real experience of a Galileo facing excommunication and perhaps death for the sake of his ideas, then it is not as romantic. If we are considering the experience of Albert Einstein who couldn't get a position as a research assistant anywhere in Europe because of his unconventional character, and who spent several years doing odd jobs until the publication of his special theory of relativity, then we are talking of real frustration and misery. In a child, these tendencies may come out in ways disturbing to conventional school order. Fadely and Hosler describe one child whose creativity was especially disruptive:

> He had been diagnosed as hyperactive, of course, and he was. He had also had the privilege of being diagnosed as "dyslexic" which had made him somewhat of a hero about the house in that the parents felt he had some dread disease from which he might recover only after a great deal of time and then only partially. This had been effective, at least, in assuring his parents' solicitous cooperation so that he could engage in his favorite pastimes of building things, painting a large dinosaur on the bathroom wall colorfully done in his mother's favorite lipstick, and leaving the family cat in a homemade rocket slated for blastoff sometime in the spring. . . . Gerald did win first prize for his Halloween creation in the form of a space robot with magnificently arranged blinking lights and whirling objects placed all about and manipulated from inside. The morning he wore it to school, he was not allowed on the bus, whereupon his mother took him to school with robot in arm. However, before he entered the school he was able to put on his creation and enter the building, terrorizing the entire kindergarten class just prior to their "show and tell" period which he disrupted by entering the room presumably by mistake. The larger part of the morning he sat in the principal's office buzzing and blinking the school secretary into distraction until the principal returned from an early morning meeting in the central office. But, he did get first prize for his Halloween costume, notwithstanding the havoc caused by his arrival in the community sometime that morning.[22]

This is not an uncommon type of happening when one is working with creative children. As far as helping them come to understand their own risk-taking tendencies, reading biography on creative people can be helpful. When creative children come to realize that many of the most creative people in history were considered to be at least a little bit "bonkers" by most of their contemporaries, it can relieve some of the personal stress.

In addition to being social risk takers, creative people usually need a rather special double-edged relationship to other people.[23]

One side of this is a tendency to be loners, needing their solitude to focus on their ideas and avoiding the limitations placed on their perspectives by social conventions of the wider society. The other side is the need for a few close, supportive friends. Sometimes it is a relationship in which they lean heavily on a few other people to underwrite their work. Sometimes it is more a mutual relationship of creators sharing ideas and encouraging each other. Some of the most creatively productive times in history have occurred when a number of creators have worked in close collaboration. This was true of the group of sixteenth century playwrights in which Shakespeare participated. This was true of the group of European scientists including Bohr, Rutherford, Planck, Poincare, Curie, and Einstein who were in close contact in the early part of this century. It was true of the artists who gathered around Gertrude Stein in Paris. It was true of the Bloomsbury group that gathered around Virginia Woolf in London. Creative children often show these tendencies toward very selective social relationships and, if they are lucky, have a few close, supportive friends.

In this section on creativity, I have referenced a number of sources of ideas for encouraging creativity. None of these sources provide a definitive answer to the need. That is probably not possible. Creativity is both the most distinctly human quality of man and also man's greatest challenge. If the process of creativity were exactly programmable like a computer, we would have been well on our way to accomplishing this by now, in which case all of the tricky issues that plague men's minds would have found ultimate solutions. Some areas of scientific understanding are so well mapped out that creative solutions may derive from computer programs. For example factor-analytic solutions in psychology are sometimes unanticipated and suggest a new theoretical perspective. These solutions, however, derive from preconceptions of the way a problem could be studied and interpretations of the results derived. It is men's minds that make computerized, creative solutions possible, not the other way around. This being the case, we may never get inside the creative process enough to accomplish it mechanically. Guidelines to creativity are probably inherently unsatisfactory to the knowledgeable.

Perhaps when encouraging creativity in children, it is more important to be observant of their behavior than to follow some prescribed curriculum. The aspects of creativity I have mentioned would be good guidelines for making observations. One should notice when children are making unusual perceptions about the world around them and try to make use of these perceptions. When a child raises questions and sees problems over issues that other children don't, a teacher should consider whether there is legitimacy or educational merit in pursuing the issues. When a child reveals sensitive, personal insights, these must be protected from ridicule. A child who goes beyond information as given to see patterns and connections on his own may be playing at the core of creativity. When a child takes a chance of seeming odd in his insistence on going his own way, we need to help him realize that he is not alone in this predicament. When a creative child is somewhat socially reserved, or has just a few close friends who are similarly creative, we should see this as part of a personally important pattern of adaptation.

REFERENCES

1. Harnadek, A. *Spatial Perception*. Pacific Grove, Calif.: Midwest Publications, 1979; Black, H., and Black, S. *Figural Analogies*. Pacific Grove, Calif.: Midwest Publications, 1981.
2. Beckman, L. The use of block design subtest of the WISC as identifying instrument for spatial children. In Gallagher, J. *Gifted Children*. Jerusalem: Kolleck and Son, Ltd., 1979.
3. Laycock, M. and Watson, G. *The Fabric of Mathematics*. Hayward, Calif.: Activity Resources Company, 1975.
4. Nuffield Mathematics Project. *Shape and Size*. New York: John Wiley, 1972.
5. Bannatyne, A. *Language, Reading and Learning Disabilities*. Springfield, Ill.: Charles C Thomas, Publishers, 1971, pp. 394-398; Fadely, J., and Hosler, V. *Understanding the Alpha Child at Home and School*. Springfield, Ill.: Charles C Thomas, Publisher, 1979, p. 115.
6. Getzels, J.W., and Jackson, P.W. The highly intelligent and the highly creative adolescent. In Vernon, P.E. *Creativity*. New York: Penguin Books, 1970, pp. 189-202.
7. Callahan, C. *Developing Creativity in the Gifted and Talented*. Reston, Virginia: Council for Exceptional Children, 1978.
8. The Burdick Group. *Creativity: The Human Resource*. San Francisco: Standard Oil Company, 1980, p. 8.
9. Allison, L. *Blood and Guts: A Working Guide to Your Own Little Insides*. Boston: Little, Brown and Co., 1976.
10. Einstein, A. and Infeld, L. *The Evolution of Physics*. New York: Simon and Schuster, 1938, p. 92.

11. Getzels, J., and Csikszentmihalyi, M. *The Creative Vision*. New York: John Wiley, 1976.
12. Parnes, S., Noller, R., and Biondi, A. *Guide to Creative Action*. New York: Charles Scribner's Sons, 1977.
13. Wallas, G. The art of thought. In Vernon, P.E. *Creativity*. New York: Penguin Books, 1970, pp. 94-95.
14. *Ibid.*, pp. 96-97.
15. Ornstein, R. *The Psychology of Consciousness*. New York: Harcourt, Brace, Jovanovich, 1977.
16. Antrobus, J., Dement, W., and Fisher, C. Patterns of dreaming and dream recall: an EEG study. *Journal of Abnormal and Social Psychology, 69*:244-252, 1964.
17. Singer, J. *The Inner World of Daydreaming*. New York: Harper and Row, 1975; Samuels, M., and Samuels, N. *Seeing with the Mind's Eye*. New York: Random House, 1975.
18. The Burdick Group, *op. cit.*
19. The Burdick Group, *op. cit.*
20. Gordon, W.J.J. and Poze, T. *The Art of the Possible*. Cambridge, Mass.: SES Associates, 1976; Williams, F. *Classroom Ideas for Encouraging Thinking and Feeling*. Buffalo, N.Y.: DOK Publications, Inc., 1970.
21. Barron, F. *Creativity and Psychological Health*. Princeton, N.J.: Van Nostrand, 1963.
22. Fadely and Hosler, *op. cit.*, pp. 120-121.
23. Lasswell, H. The social setting of creativity. In Anderson, H.H. *Creativity and Its Cultivation*. New York: Harper Brothers, 1959.

Chapter 9

SOCIAL ENVIRONMENT AND
SOCIAL LEARNING

A NEEDED SPECIAL ENVIRONMENT

A LONG history of research, which was reviewed in Chapter 6, indicates a relationship between spatial ability and certain personality characteristics. It has been found that children who possess considerable spatial-mechanical ability but more limited verbal ability are often characterized by an introverted, independent, socially reserved personality. The cognitive style of these children requires the integration of large amounts of information into complex gestalt systems. This mental work necessitates a carefully controlled relationship to the outer world. The integration of new information into such systems requires time and effort and can easily be interfered with by stimulus overload. Communicating complex ideas to other people can be slow and laborious. It is important for parents and teachers to be aware of this personality style and to be prepared to relate to it in an appropriate manner.

As a part of this personality style, spatial children often possess a sensitive reactivity to their social environment. If not handled properly, this reactivity can be destructive to the child. For example it is known that introverted children perform learning tasks at a much more satisfactory level when they are in situations of low arousal. Michael Eysenck has found that, in addition to having more memory problems than other people, they are especially affected by the degree of activation they feel. In verbal fluency tasks ("name all the animal names you can think of"), Eysenck found that whereas extroverts perform at a higher level when they feel pressured or aroused, it was just the opposite for introverts. They performed at a lower level when aroused.[1]

Related results were obtained in a study by George Thompson and Clarence Hunnicutt. They were interested in seeing how blame or praise would affect the work of introverts and extroverts. People were given a set of six tests in which they were presented with a long series of random numbers. They were asked to quickly cross out one given number (say seven) in the whole series of numbers. After completion of each test, the tester looked carefully at each paper and then, irrespective of the actual performance, placed a *P* for poor work (blame) or a *G* for good work (praise) on the test paper. The purpose was to see how this arbitrarily assigned blame or praise would affect subsequent performance. The researchers found that extroverted people achieved their best performance under conditions of blame and introverted people achieved their best performance under conditions of praise.[2]

The exact psychological dynamics behind the effects of praise and blame can only be guessed at. Perhaps, under conditions of indiscriminant praise, the work of the socially responsive extroverts became sloppy, while the work of the socially independent introverts remained task-committed. Under conditions of continual blame, the introverts may have become stressed and confused by a task they thought was quite simple, while the extroverts become motivated by the social pressure to improve and by a higher level of arousal.

Whatever the explanation for these results, the Eysenck findings and the Thompson and Hunnicutt findings point to the need for establishing a special kind of environment for introverted spatial children. Nonarousing environments are sometimes difficult to achieve in school settings, but it would be negligent to fail to make the attempt when working with spatial children. The time pressures that children get subjected to are often unnecessary and have little to do with the more profound and creative thought processes.

Testing is sometimes a problem in this regard. Although all children need the experience of taking tests, test taking is too often an unnecessarily disturbing experience. One of the principal aims of testing should be to teach children how to alleviate the stress associated with testing.

The techniques for emphasizing praise rather than blame are readily available to any teacher. Most approaches to behavior modification are based on this principle. It is just a matter of emphasis as to whether a teacher focuses on failures or focuses on successes in attempting to encourage the work of students. Even at the beginning stages of student work, when mistakes are abundant, it is possible to limit the scope of evaluation and to deliberately find those limited aspects of accomplishment for which a student can be lauded. If there are doubts about the possibilities of emphasizing positive reinforcement in the classroom, any good textbook on behavior modification could be consulted.

An objection might be raised that rather than adjusting school environments to the needs of children, we should be helping children adjust to school environments. To some extent, children need to become adaptable to a variety of environments. They will be faced with a variety of environments throughout their lives. The opposing argument is that, to the extent that a slow, meticulous, deliberative cognitive style is essential to the best work of spatial children, it is a mistake to force them to adjust to environments that undermine their unusual capabilities.

LEARNING CREATIVE RESPONSE TO THE SOCIAL ENVIRONMENT

It was noted in Chapter 6 that spatial children may have difficulties in relating socially to other people and that this may lead to a degree of social isolation. To the extent that introversion is an aspect of the natural personality style of the child, teachers and parents should never attempt to prevent the child from seeking appropriate solitude in carrying out his productive work. Nevertheless, social isolation and social ineffectiveness are sometimes experienced as an uncomfortable problem to the child. Just as it would not do to force the child out of his most comfortable cognitive style, it would also not be appropriate to ignore the social discomfort.

The key to working with the delicate dilemma is to use an approach to developing social skills that is nonthreatening to children, in which they will participate without pressure or coercion.

A program developed by the Center for Theatre Techniques in Education would appear to meet this criterion. Mary Hunter Wolf, a theater innovator, realized that some of the basic skills learned in theatrical training can be important to anyone in the development of social effectiveness. She developed methods of using theater training techniques with school children. In this programming, training techniques are modified so that they start with the most elementary levels of development and with activities that are as completely nonthreatening to the child as possible. Children gradually move toward participation in social interactions that they would not have thought themselves capable of prior to participation in the program.

Having had the opportunity to evaluate a component of this program, I was able to collect information that may indicate that it is particularly appropriate for use with spatial children. Since the program usually operates on a completely voluntary basis, one of the points of interest is the extent to which various types of children choose to participate after an initial exposure. In this particular component, information was available on the spatial and nonverbal abilities of children, on the creative abilities of children, and on the achievement skills of children. Spatial, nonverbal abilities were assessed through the Differential Aptitude Tests, creative ability through the Torrance Tests of Creative Thinking, and achievement skills through the Iowa Tests of Basic Skills.

From this information, it was possible to determine test score patterns for each child prior to exposure to the program. Most particularly, it was determined which of the three skill areas was the greatest strength for a given child. From this comparison, it was found that the student whose personal strength was in spatial, nonverbal ability was predominant among those children who chose to remain in the program after an initial year of exposure.

The most complete description of the theater techniques program is in a book called *Bananas and Fifty-Four Other Varieties*.[3] The goals of the program as described in this book are as follows:

> Community: refers to the first phase of the work — establishing a learning community — so that every student is able to contribute comfortably to the learning process.

> Concentration: refers to the student's discovery of a learning style which can be focused and called upon readily.

> Imagination: is the inner workings of each student's personal responses and can be a great source of commitment to problem solving.

> Environment: is the awareness and utilization of all forms of space — self and sensory equipment, demographic and topographic, the community and the world — as places for living.

It is not possible to give a description of the program that is both adequate and brief. I can only describe three activities and recommend that *Bananas and Fifty-Four Other Varieties* be consulted for further details. The activities consistently are arranged from those involving simple essentials to those having a more complex structure.

This means that the activities move from a low risk level and proceed to more challenging and involving variations and combinations.

Classes often begin with the *Introduction Game*. Seated in a circle, students give their names and some additional fact about themselves (favorite toy, occupation when they grow up, etc.). An appropriate gesture or motion accompanies the fact (steering motion for airplane pilot, etc.). Each child takes a turn introducing all the preceding students to the group and then adds his own introduction. In this way all names, facts, and motions are repeated many times as they go around the group. By the time the game is finished, each child knows the name of all others in the group. It is generally a discovery for the child that those with the largest number of facts to remember toward the end of the game do extremely well because reinforcement has been provided by repetition, by association of facts and gestures, and by accepting assistance easily without sense of failure. This can be an especially important discovery for the spatial child who often has problems with memory for details. Another general benefit is that the individual is looked at intently by all members of the group. This simple experience, which under other circumstances might well be loaded with self-consciousness, becomes familiar and loses its tension.

Other identification techniques are used as well; students line up quickly in order by height, by shades of clothing, by house numbers, and so forth. In these activities, students learn to change positions lightly and easily and to arrange themselves into groups. The individual's concentration is totally addressed to performing the operation as rapidly as possible rather than on self-conscious thoughts. At the same time, the activity involves having the child's characteristics focused on and accepted in the group order.

At a more advanced level, an activity called *Circle Story* might be used. This is a good way for students to begin work on dramatic content and to experience how imaginative material from the individual can be accepted and developed in the group context. One student begins a story with one sentence, several words, or one word. Thereafter, each student continues and adds to the story in the same manner until all have contributed, and there is a sense that the story is complete. The circle story can then be refined. The instructor can ask questions that highlight principles of story development. This might include definition of character, situation, reasons for certain occurrences, motive for certain actions, relationships of people, role of characters, and sequence of events. This is good exercise in social analysis and is especially valuable for children who are not particularly adept at social comprehension.

A circle story may then be performed. During the rehearsal process, the students discuss human feelings as portrayed by actors in the dramatic context, and they make refinements accordingly. One student serves as director while others work in small groups to develop the music and sound effects, sets, visual effects, and the acting and movement. They learn about timing, plot, characterization, and audience reaction. A final performance that integrates these elements may be recorded on videotape.

Circle story starts with the simplest, most nonthreatening format, yet it can lead to the most complex social analysis. Since the purpose is development of social understanding and creative group process, not formal performance, it is essential to retain an easygoing, nonjudgmental atmosphere throughout the activity. If some kind of performance does result from the circle story, the emphasis should not be on formal presentation, but rather on showing what the group has created. Spatial children might be the last to get involved in a program that has the purpose of theatrical performance. Yet, they often find this relaxed, playful approach to social learning to be enjoyable.

These sample activities don't present a full sense of the total theater techniques program. The book *Bananas and Fifty-Four Other Varieties* should be consulted for that purpose.

SOCIAL-PSYCHOLOGICAL EXPLORATION

It was noted in Chapter 6 that when the spatial child suffers some emotional difficulty, he is likely to go in the direction of a withdrawn pulling away from social relations. In the less common and extreme cases, a child may reach the level of outright hostility toward others and exhibit aggressive behavior. It is best that some provision be made in the school curriculum for helping children achieve a degree of self-understanding.

Although the research gives no clear guidance in establishing such a curriculum, the personality characteristics typical in the spatial child might suggest that an exploratory-cognitive approach to self-understanding is more likely to be valuable to the child than a therapeutic-dependency approach. To the extent that the spatial child tends to be independent and self-sufficient in character, the child is likely to resist therapeutic approaches that depend on authoritative pronouncements or on submitting to dependency on some authoritative person. Instead, the child needs the opportunity to study the meaning and function of emotional experience. Attempts at indoctrination into some version of therapeutic philosophy like Freudian psychology, humanistic psychology, or behavioral psychology would seem to the child as conventionally restrictive as learning grammar for the sake of learning grammar.

If the child's own emotional experience can be used as the basis for a general creative exploration of man's psychological experience, then the emotional experience of the child can be given positive significance rather than a negative significance as something requiring therapy. The fact that Freud's own emotional experience formed the basis for his understanding of others, and the fact that this has been true for almost all great psychological thinkers, can be used as the starting point for creative exploration. Children who are very independent and nonconforming in social character would tend to appreciate the creative method of Freud, Jung, Maslow, or Skinner, while they might resent attempts by others to force interpretation of their own behavior into the terms of any one legitimized system.

The approach to be used with a group of children depends on the age level. For children below age ten or twelve, the best approach would involve reading children's stories that give concrete examples of children dealing with different kinds of problems. There are many good children's storybooks along this line. A good bibliography on such material is provided in Joan Fassler's book, *Helping Children Cope.*[4]

For children above twelve, a more academic approach to investigation could be used. To have a class in which psychological and social issues are explored would be good. Some of the best material would be biographical and autobiographical readings on the lives of people who have made important contributions to psychology. Children can become familiar with the experiences that led psychologists to develop their ideas. Psychological investigation can thus take its place within the realm of human experience, and students can see the possibility of using experiences of their own as the basis for achieving a personal psychological understanding. They can also become critics of the conclusions of established psychology and, thus, retain the feeling of security in the independence of their perspectives.

When working in this area with either older or younger children, it is important to allow self-insights to emerge spontaneously. Pressing children to share their experiences before they feel ready to do so on their own initiative is likely to be threatening and to close off later opportunities to share. It is also important to allow the child's own self-knowledge and self-control to be the most important basis for adaptation. A sense of control over one's situation is one of the best indicators of the adjustment and well-being of a person. For a spatial child, this might be more important than for other children. Therapeutic work done with the spatial child should be initiated from the assumption that when the child is sincerely giving attention to a problem, the child himself is the best source of knowledge about the problem and most capable of deciding on a course of action that will lead to a solution. The most important thing is to set up an environment in which the child can feel comfortable and unthreatened as he gropes toward knowledge and toward important decisions.

TIME PLANNING

Sometimes spatial children have difficulty with the time and sequence planning that is often required for reaching significant goals. They may accurately see accomplishments in terms of the ingredients involved, but not see the accomplishments so well in terms of how the ingredients are put together over a period of time. Time charting is one approach to developing insights about sequencing. At the beginning of a student project, a teacher can have students think of all the tasks involved in carrying out the project. The students can then create some type of time-line chart in which the tasks are sequenced in an appropriate manner. As students begin carrying out the tasks in the sequence, there should be an emphasis on recording each accomplishment and encouraging students to see each accomplishment as a valuable step in reaching the desired goal. The students learn that important accomplishments in life are usually the result of a series of smaller accomplishments. This will be especially helpful to spatial children who sometimes see things in terms of their simultaneous ingredients, rather than in terms of a sequence of steps.

REFERENCES

1. Eysenck, M.W. Extroversion, arousal, and retrieval from semantic memory. *Journal of Personality, 42*:319-331, 1974.
2. Thompson, G.C., and Hunnicutt, C.W. The effects of repeated praise or blame on the work achievement of introverts and extroverts. *Journal of Educational Psychology, 35*:256-266, 1944.
3. Grenough, M., Marshall, B., McGuire, L., O'Rourke, K. and Spector, P. *Bananas and Fifty-Four Other Varieties*. Stratford, Conn.: Center for Theatre Techniques in Education, 1980.
4. Fassler, J. *Helping Children Cope*. New York: The Free Press, 1978.

Chapter 10

LANGUAGE ARTS

ACHIEVING MEANING AND PURPOSE
IN LANGUAGE ARTS

Too often teachers and parents are misled by behavioral psychologists into looking at language as a purely technical process. We are led to believe that if we understand the technical aspects of reading, approach them in an appropriate manner, and provide some encouragement to the child, all problems can be overcome. Under this influence, teachers begin to act as if they were operating an assembly line in which this skill and that skill are mounted to a frame as it passes down the assembly line. Teaching becomes a skill bookkeeping chore in which the accumulation of skills is an end in itself. We begin to act as if language arts should be pursued for their own sake, for the teacher's bookkeeping sake, or for the sake of a parent's pride. This approach may work for many children, but for spatial children, it is likely to be a serious error.

The motivational side of language is especially important for spatial children. Unlike many other children, they have little motivation to pursue language study for its own sake. Being inclined to take in the full sensory depth and breadth of the world around them, the very idea of spending hours scanning with one's eyes along rows of small black shapes called letters is antithetical to what life is about for these children. The repulsiveness of the teacher's demand to narrow one's sensory field of intake to such boring "book-scapes" causes the child to meander in his reading behavior and to fill his mind with interesting daydreams far removed from the content of the reading. Failure to tie language learning to the things that are fascinating to the child are bound to render all other technically grounded teaching relatively ineffective. For the spatial child, language will always be a vehicle, perhaps a difficult one, for achieving other purposes.

Fadely and Hosler have listed some of the less inspiring reasons for learning to read, which often get communicated to a child either

197

directly or through attitude and teaching practice.[1]

1. One learns to read to become literate.
2. One learns to read because that is what one goes to school for.
3. One learns to read in order to obtain a passing grade so one can pass to the next grade to learn to read better.
4. One learns to read because it is fun to read.
5. One learns to read because parents expect one to and because personal worth is determined by how well one reads.
6. One learns to read because learning is the work of children.
7. One learns to read so that one can become a productive member of the community.
8. One learns to read so one can get a good job.
9. One learns to read because in order to be successful one has to be able to read.
10. One learns to read because it makes one smart.

For many children, these reasons for learning to read present no problem. Many children can accept learning to read for its own sake or for the sake of some brand of social conformity. For the spatial child who will have more difficulty with language and whose mind may be wandering off into the broader meanings of life, these do not provide sufficient motivation. For these children, language skill acquisition must always be tied to highly motivating content — content that derives in some way from the child's own interests. Fadely and Hosler have also listed some of the nobler reasons for learning to use language — reasons that when kept in mind in curriculum planning are more likely to inspire the child.[2]

1. Words convey history and history establishes our place in time, our meaning as a culture, our heritage, and future. Words bring the past and the future into full view when neither can exist without language and words. More importantly, language symbols, verbal and nonverbal, provide the means of communicating information and ideas. Upon such ideas our minds can grow into expanded awareness and being.
2. Words provide an abstract way of learning about the feelings of others, of their hopes, ideas, and concerns.
3. Words provide the means of filing, in retrievable form, our past experience and future dreams. Language and words define our own history, our personal place in time and space.
4. Words provide an extensive data bank of information that can be used to evaluate, to elaborate, to synthesize, and to create new information and ideas.
5. Words provide the mechanical means to travel from practical to abstract and back again to practical.

6. Words provide the means to test the environment surrounding us, to learn of its nature, to find ways to live in harmony with the world about us.

7. Words and books provide the means of giving each of us independence in personal growth for we can seek out information that is important to us as individuals. Words bring the thoughts and knowledge of great teachers and philosophers to us as if the person were there.

8. Words and books open the storehouses of knowledge to us all.

9. Words bring the potential for personal meaning.

As long as these nobler purposes for reading and writing are kept at the heart of our teaching, we will have a higher probability of turning spatial children on to the effective use of language.

The place of motivation in the use of language was brought home to me most forcefully several years ago when I helped organize a teaching program in a street academy. This was a school for high school dropouts. More properly, the students in this school should have been called "push-outs." Other schools had essentially given up on them as hopeless. When the teachers in the street academy attempted to get these students to relate to any ordinary reading material, there was a complete show of reading incompetence and disinterest. How the students had made it to the high school level was beyond imagination.

Fortunately, a teacher at the street academy had the good sense to bring in a number of copies of *The Autobiography of Malcolm X*. Most of the students in the school were inner-city black children. Their identification with Malcolm X was immediate. Without encouragement or reward from the teachers, the copies of Malcolm X circulated throughout the student body. Most of the students read the book from cover to cover. This was a book several times longer than anything most had read before. The students were recalling details from the book months later. Some of the students in the school were spatial children, and some of these children were most active in this educational happening.

Alexander Bannatyne echoed this theme as the foundation for all of his more technical curriculum recommendations.[3]

> With boys and girls seven years of age and over, I have found it useful to encourage the child to select a theme or topic in which he or she is extremely interested. This is used as a basis for most of the lessons and on occasion may even be developed into a work project which, of course, will involve a great deal of spelling, writing, and reading. Pirates, racing cars,

pop music groups and even science topics such as geology are the topics of subject matter which might be used. One intelligent high school boy, a poor speller who aimed to be a geologist, read and wrote reams on rocks and minerals. Even though he required much help in reading advanced books, his progress was probably much more rapid than it would have been using traditional readers.

In the following sections of this chapter on language arts curriculum, I have collected a number of teaching techniques that are consistent with the learning style of the spatial child and that at the same time allow for the creative incorporation of the child's interests and experiences. Whatever the technical methods used, a teacher who keeps each child's interests and experiences central to the teaching process cannot go far wrong in working with spatial children. In the words of Fadely and Hosler, the first need of these children is "to learn to speak of one's feelings, to find verbal expression for all of the sensitivity and awareness that runs rampant through the mind . . . These children require much opportunity to talk, to express in some consistent manner what they feel and know."[4]

LANGUAGE EXPERIENCE APPROACHES

Research on the processes involved in learning to read has in the past tended to focus on one major issue. Should reading be introduced through phonetic principles emphasizing word recognition, or should it be introduced through whole word principles that emphasize the meaningfulness and experiential significance of language? In most simplistic terms, the phoneticist would start by associating the letters *d, o,* and *g* with certain spoken sounds and then teach children how to connect the sounds to arrive at the association between the written word *dog* and the spoken word *dog.* The whole-word teacher would start with the spoken word *dog* along with pictures of dogs and then introduce children to the fact that the whole written word associated with this concept is *dog.*

Both the phoneticists and the whole-word teachers will probably groan at the simplicity of this explanation. Nevertheless, it wouldn't serve my purpose to go into the finer points of the two approaches. More important is the fact that most researchers and teachers have come to the conclusion that both approaches can play an important role in teaching children to read. It is important to find ways to use both in a coordinated manner. Both approaches involve special techniques that are important for the spatial child. In this section, the whole-word approach will be presented first because it deals most directly with the motivational issues that are central to the reading difficulties of the spatial child and because it fits most closely the cognitive style of the spatial child. In the next section, I will present a phonetic approach that also fits the cognitive style of the spatial child.

The whole-word approach begins with the language experience of the child. One starts by having a child express himself in a variety of ways using his own vocabulary; this expression is then used as a basis for teaching reading. A teacher might start by having children tell short stories of interesting things that have happened to them. Initially, these stories could be tape-recorded. Then stories can either be written on the chalk board or typed by the teacher. Various words can be picked out from the stories so that the children in a class can come to connect each word to its place in a story and experience repeated recognition and pronunciation of the words as whole, meaningful entities. Children can copy their stories into storybooks they construct so that repeated writing of their own vocabulary can lead to faster word recognition.

As a child develops some sight vocabulary, a teacher can increase the complexity of the process by suggesting new words that might be used in interesting ways in the stories. Interesting and varied stories can be created by having several children cooperate in the creation of a story, perhaps in a manner similar to the circle story described in Chapter 9. Also, children can be helped toward more complete story telling patterns that include introductions, descriptions of characters, situational development, and conclusions. Some simple outlining could be introduced to help children structure their more complex stories. One key to the whole-word approach is the use of personal experience to enhance motivation. The other key is the repeated use of words and rereading of stories so that the recognition of individual words becomes fast and automatic.

Fadely and Hosler suggest that because the spatial child is more sensitive to the gestalt, figural nature of words than to the actual spelling details, it is sometimes helpful to have them focus on this.[5] Children can outline the shape of words. This focusing on shape can be an aid in both word recognition and in spelling. Another aid that

Fadely and Hosler recommend is having children read when they are singing. Many spatial children enjoy singing. The repeated reading of words used in songs will contribute to recognition skills.

It should be recognized that there is a need to establish a basic sight vocabulary (quick recognition of high frequency words), such as that provided in the Dolch system.[6] However, even that should be done through the language experience approach. If it is noticed that certain high frequency words don't seem to be coming into a child's own story production, these words should be introduced and the child should be encouraged to find ways of using the words.

After connecting basic sight vocabulary to the child's experience, flash cards containing these words can be separated into boxes according to their parts of speech. This can create an initial awareness of the parts of speech and also allows words to be used in sentence structure games. Children can be shown a sentence with a very common structure, such as article–noun–verb–preposition–article–noun (e.g. "The dog jumped over the rope."). By randomly selecting new words from the appropriate parts of speech boxes to replace the words in the original sentence, children can make up new sentences that have the same structure but a different, and sometimes strange, meaning. An equivalent sentence to the example above might be the following: "A basketball barked in the mouse."

This kind of sentence game can give a feeling for the structure of language, a feeling for the flexibility of language, and a feeling for the way language can be used in imaginative and fanciful ways. Could the idea of a basketball barking in a mouse be used by a child to create an imaginative story?. For children who enjoy playing around with the general structure of things and who also enjoy using their imaginations, this type of game can provide motivation.

DEALING WITH PHONETIC INCONSISTENCY

Since the spatial child tends to be a holistic synthesizer of information rather than a detailed, linear processor, this leads to sequential memory problems of all sorts. Sequencing is basic to language, and this is one reason why spatial children can have extensive difficulties with language. In the English language, sequencing difficulties are compounded by the fact that English is not a very phonetic language. In other words, the rules that guide the relationship between the written word and the spoken word are full of inconsistencies. This is a problem whichever direction one is going, from the spoken word to the written, or the written to the spoken.

When going from the spoken to the written word, as in a spelling test, the oddities that must be memorized abound. Sounding out a word like *beautiful* doesn't begin to lead to the officially recognized spelling. In addition to the letter sequence *eau* being very rare in English, phonetically the *eau* might be expected to be a simple *u* (butiful). Even after the child knows that there is an *e*, an *a* and a *u* involved, it could still be *eua, uae, uea, aeu,* or *aue.* Who could even guess at such devious, verbose nonsense?

When going from the written word to the spoken word, the problems similarly abound. For example these seven words all rhyme:

To	Grew
Through	Too
Moo	True
Two	

Yet each contains a different spelling for the same phoneme. As if having seven or more spellings for the same phoneme were not bad enough, the same spelling can be associated with several phonemes. Vowels have several different pronunciations, and even a complex letter group like *ough* is pronounced one way in *through*, another way in *though*, and still a third way in *enough*.

This apparent chaos in English spelling has caused many educators to abandon the attempts to teach reading through phonics. Trying to pretend that there is a system when there isn't can be more confusing than helpful to some children. Learning phonetic rules that are not really rules just adds to the information load for a child. This is especially problematic for spatial children who have difficulty dealing with large amounts of detailed information, who spend their time looking for the systematic and patterned aspects of information, and who are perplexed when they can't find any.

These problems do not necessarily mean that we should abandon phonetic instruction. When rule-based patterns can be used in instruction, this can reduce the information load on a child. Facts can be reproduced on the basis of consistent relationships. This is true in a more phonetic language like Spanish. If a phonetic approach is used in teaching reading to the spatial child, it must be based on some method that makes the language phonetic. Several systems have been invented to do this. Among them is one created by Alexander Bannatyne and called the Psycholinguistic Color System.[7] "In the Psycholinguistic Color System, only the seventeen vowel phonemes are color-coded, and this is done in such a way that the name of the color itself indicates the sound of the vowel phoneme. For example, the phoneme /ee/ as in the word green is colored green and all the graphemes which are spellings of the sound /ee/ are also colored green, e.g. field, receipt, bean." Bannatyne has used his system extensively with spatial children in order to make the English language phonetic for the introduction of reading.[8]

The same idea of creating phonetic consistency was followed in the creation of the Initial Teaching Alphabet.[9] In this system, new letter shapes similar to the usual ones have been created to represent each distinct phoneme. When children first learn to read, all materials are in the new alphabet. Initial decoding is simplified. Once a child has achieved rapid decoding in the Initial Teaching Alphabet, there is a switch to the regular alphabet. The assumption is that the similarities between the appearance of words in the Initial Teaching Alphabet and their appearance in the regular alphabet is great enough so that the child will find it easy to switch from one to the other. The ease with which this switch is made is not so well established.[10]

The advantage of a color-coded system, such as that created by Bannatyne, is that the regular spelling of words can be used at the same time that the words are phonetically coded. Children can become sensitive to the correct spelling of a word at the same time they are learning its pronunciation. The switch for the child is when the color coding is dropped. This switch is less a problem because the spelling remains the same throughout.

The most widely used color-coded system has been created by Caleb Gattegno and is called *Words-In-Color*. Gattegno insists that any child who can speak has already mastered a most complex system of relationships between sounds and meanings. If reading is approached in a natural way, it is simply a matter of extending that mastery to a visual code. In teaching reading, color-coded charts are used to connect the natural speech of a child to the construction of written words. This is done in a flowing way intended to correspond to the linear sequencing of natural speech.

Writing is the codification of spoken speech, and reading its reverse process. What is written is nothing if it is not speech. How do we bridge the gap between the two types of speech? This is the problem of teaching reading. . . . Before anyone can reach spoken speech, he must already have access to meanings or he could retain nothing. . . . And once we have a general access to meaning, then we can put different labels on it, and the labels will stick to the meaning. . . . Given this, there is very little to do in order to go from spoken speech to written speech. . . . Comprehension then follows from the capacity to utter the signs seen, as words but with the flow of speech and the melody of the language, the capacity to attach the appropriate meanings to all the words uttered.[11]

The approach has proven helpful to a wide variety of children who have difficulty with reading.[12] Through its logical and consistent structure, it would most certainly be helpful to spatial children. There doesn't seem to be any information on the relative merits of the Bannatyne color-coded system and the Gattegno system. One or the other could be used depending on the relative availability of materials and teacher training in either system.

SPELLING

Spatial children often have difficulty with the recall of any detailed information that cannot be reconstructed from patterns or systems of knowledge. Because English spelling is so nonphonetic, it is one of the chief memory problem areas. This has led to the anomaly of the very bright child who is atrocious at spelling. Bannatyne has observed that "Many boys who have learned to read at a comparatively late age have, through sheer reasoning ability, obtained a place in an academically inclined school, and while from the conceptualizing point of view they can hold their own, their work is marred by extremely irregular spelling."[13]

In recommending an approach to this problem, Bannatyne stresses that repetition should be central to any spelling program. The memory weakness requires that spelling be overlearned. A limited number of words should be focused on each week (approximately 12). The words under study should be continually used throughout the week. They can be put in complete sentences; the more humorous the better. In this repeated use of words, correct information on the spelling of a word should be immediately available to the child, and feedback on mistakes should be immediate. In this way, practice of incorrect spelling is avoided, as is frustration. Methods of correcting mistakes should avoid implying inadequacy in the child or punishing the child for his weakness.

Beyond these general recommendations, Bannatyne sees a phonetically based approach to spelling as being most valuable for the spatial child. This goes along with his phonetic, color-coded approach to initial reading. Spelling should involve a careful training in oral articulation of a word and the way its parts fit together as a pattern of sounds. The articulation can then be matched with the visual configuration broken into visual parts.

> If difficult words are broken into syllables, the child will be able to see that a long word is really only a series of quite manageable short "bits" which can themselves be strung together in much the same way as letters are. Moreover, the child will come to understand that the "bits" as syllables have their own conventional spellings and can be arranged and rearranged in various sequences to form many other words. This can be the basis of several word games, especially if little cards with syllables, prefixes, roots and suffixes are printed with a fiber pen, e.g., how many words can you make by adding prefixes and suffixes to the root "tract"? (contract, extract, tractor, tractable, retractability, intractable, etc.).[14]

Age-appropriate dictionaries should be available, and for reinforcing particularly difficult words, Bannatyne recommends having the child keep a notebook of words that he commonly misspells. Letter sequencing should be emphasized because this is often central to the child's difficulty. Bannatyne recommends combining the visual, the vocal-auditory, and the manual approaches to sequencing. This might involve constructing words from letter blocks and naming out loud the letters as they are placed in the left-to-right order. It is important that words be spelled from beginning to end so that automatic sequencing is developed. Never let the child begin a word in the middle. Figure tracing of words in large cursive letters can reinforce sequencing. Syllable cards can also be used in sequencing so that words come to be seen as sequences of syllables as well as sequences of letters.

Because of his emphasis on a phonetic approach, Bannatyne discourages commonly used oral memorization methods. He said, "words must be phonetically sounded out,"[15] not simply spelled automatically without giving thought to the sounds. Fadely and Hosler, on the other hand, emphasizing the holistic nature of the thinking of the spatial child, recommend exactly the opposite approach. They claim that oral sequencing of letters corresponds to holistic perception.[16]

> Since he has so much difficulty remembering specific phonetic sounds and integrating them, the phonetic approach is somewhat useless, but if he is asked to say the letters of the word out loud, he will often recognize them. In essence, spelling the words out loud as he looks at them often aides holistic recognition. Thus, one technique which should always be tried is that of having the child say each letter out loud and to see if this assists recall and recognition. It often will.

As an extension of the whole-word approach to reading, Fadely and Hosler emphasize that spelling of words should be learned as they enter the child's reading vocabulary. Lessons in oral spelling go along with lessons in sight recognition of each new group of words. Children first learn to recognize and pronounce words, then they practice auditory spelling, and finally they practice writing words and entering them into compositions. Spelling first and writing later is considered the proper developmental approach for this type of child.

Although the Bannatyne approach and the Fadely and Hosler approach may be thought of as mutually exclusive, it doesn't have to be that way. To the extent that spelling of words can be easily derived from a logical phonetic analysis made possible by Bannatyne's color coding system, phonetic analysis can be used in spelling. On the other hand, to the extent that a given word tends to defy phonetic analysis, the spatial child can better rely on an oral holistic sequencing of letters as suggested by Fadely and Hosler. Children can be taught sensitivity to when a spelling can best be approached one way or the other and to use the best method in each situation. Using both approaches when appropriate can provide variety and help retain the interest of the child.

Perhaps the most important point is that overlearning of limited amounts of information will be most helpful for the spatial child. This can be done through either approach. While using a slow continual approach to acquiring spelling vocabulary, social support and understanding of the child's problem must always be present. If the child comes to feel inadequate, the result is likely to be avoidance rather than serious work to alleviate the problem.

Word games are of great value. Lexicon®, Junior Scrabble®, spelling bees, etc., all help, particularly if the teacher is tolerant. The child's particular problem must be brought into the open with brothers, sisters, friends, and classmates and these should all be encouraged to help sympathetically rather than to scoff. Nobody should pretend that the spelling difficulty does not exist and genuine allowances should be made for it in all games. . . . There is no substitute for motivation and serious work.[17]

LISTENING AND SPEAKING

Spatial children sometimes have a tendency to give a low level of attention to verbal information. Unless extended verbal information is highly stimulating, their minds will have a tendency to wander off into an inner daydream world of personal images. This is often the child's preferred mode of cognition. This preferred mode should not be maligned by teachers or parents. Jerome Singer has demonstrated that the world of imagery is of considerable benefit to the creative development of a person.[18]

Nevertheless, there are times when this cognitive mode is not particularly adaptive. When a child is reading, but not really attending to it, this is a waste of time. Failure to attend to instructions in classroom activities can leave the child lost. The child may even fail to attend to his own verbalizations, leaving his sentences confusing. This may involve mispronouncing individual words, using unconventional sentence organizations that seem garbled to other people, or organizing ideas in such a scrambled way that other people can't discern the intended purpose or meaning.

The other side of this problem is that even when the spatial child focuses on the content of verbal information, he will tend to form a global conception of its meaning rather than a detailed one. The child may have a good general idea of what is involved, but he won't necessarily be able to recall details without assistance.

Perhaps the starting point in working with this problem is to improve attending behavior. At the Frostig School, a game is used for this purpose. Children listen to a series of directions given by a teacher (stand up, put your right hand behind your back, step forward with your left foot, put your left hand in the air, look at the ceiling, etc.) and then try to carry out the sequence. By starting with very simple instructions and increasing the difficulty gradually, children become comfortable with the process of developing more complex attending behavior. Children sometimes enjoy turning this into a competitive game in which they challenge each other to carry out longer and longer series of instructions. Creative instructions are motivating to children, and they enable children to practice giving complicated descriptions to each other.

After improving on attending to other people, children should be involved in activities that help them attend to their own utterances. Fadely and Hosler suggest that a tape recorder can be useful. Children can practice speaking or reading into the recorder, listen to themselves, correct their own mispronunciations and garbled speech, and do repeated recordings until they feel satisfied with their own production. Two or more children can do this activity together to increase interest, to share sensitivities to speech, and to share triumphs.

> This approach is based on the child's need for ego reinforcement. Aside from the pleasure of using his own voice to reinforce his reading, he also gains a more personalized and motivating stimulus from listening to the errors on tape. The child delights in being able to correct himself and he sees real progress. This tape should be saved and the child should review the tape occasionally to assure that retention remains solid. As he makes more tapes for his file, they provide him with a continuing record of his progress throughout the year.[19]

Once there is progress in both listening and pronunciation skills, a new focus can be placed on the organization of the content of speech. For younger children show-and-tell activities can be used. Puppetry activities are valuable. Children can make their own puppets from odd materials, think up voices and personalities for their puppets, make up stories in which two or more puppets are involved, and then put on informal productions.

For older children, pretending to be radio or television commentators can achieve the same purpose. Recordings can be made of actual radio or television programs so that children can transcribe and study the organization and content of the programming. How does a commentator organize the presentation of an idea? How does he arrange the details? How is a topic closed out? Notice of these aspects in the verbalizations of people who are very effective in speaking can provide good examples for children who don't use these speech patterns automatically. Studying these ideas in relation to radio or television programs that are of high interest to a child can be intriguing. Even fascinating material depends on a learnable delivery technique.

WRITING

Two principles need to be kept in mind when teaching writing to the spatial child. First, grasp of the sequential structure of language won't come as automatically and easily as it does for most other children. Sequential structure must be focused on as an intellectual problem in itself. Second, the experience and imagination of the individual child will be the most important motivation for writing — more important than content derived from any other source. Children should be expected to collect information from other sources that relate to their interest; however, their interests will make this search worth doing.

A writing curriculum that adheres very closely to these principles is called Individual Language Arts.[20] The curriculum was developed in the Weehawken, New Jersey, Public Schools and is among those validated as effective by the United States Department of Education. The Weehawken curriculum was planned with two assumptions in mind — assumptions that correspond very closely to the principles stated above. First, "certain insights provided by linguistics, the study of language, could be translated into techniques (strategies) for improving selected aspects of writing instruction." Many of these derived techniques focus on those structure of language issues that are often most challenging to the spatial child. The second assumption was that the techniques could be "blended with a language-experience approach so that the language, experiences, feelings, and ideas of students can be used to promote motivation, precision, and control." This is the other principle most important for the spatial child. The curriculum proceeds from the understanding that a person who does much writing beyond the school experience does so —

> to express joy or happiness or gratitude,
> to voice his wonder or curiosity or compassion,
> to provide an outlet for anger or hostility,
> to verbalize anxieties or worries,
> to express friendship or personal interest,
> to express an opinion or to editorialize,
> to advance an idea or a theory or an explanation,
> to describe an event or an incident,
> to give or request information,

to apply for a job, and
to fulfill job requirements.[21]

In the Weehawken curriculum, writing activities are oganized to follow a pattern called the *communication spiral*. The spiral starts with some experience that is personally meaningful to students. This leads to discussion among students and to planning for writing. The writing is done by individuals or by groups of students. There is oral reading of compositions, discussion, and evaluation by students. Compositions may go through several improvement phases. Oral reading of all compositions is considered an essential part of the process. Through these readings, students develop a strong sense of how their compositions will be understood by others. In other words, school writing is grounded in the purpose of all good writing: to communicate effectively to others. A graphic representation of the communication spiral is given in Figure 10-1.[22]

Along with initiating writing within the context of its social purpose, the Weehawken curriculum uses linguistic concepts to focus on skills that are essential to good writing. Part of this focus on basic skills involves the development of a writing checklist for student use and a diagnostic grid sheet for teacher use. The student's writing checklist accumulates gradually as a listing of skills that the student has mastered or is near mastering. The checklist acts as a reminder of things that should be looked for in compositions. The checklist may start with one or two items so that the student isn't overloaded with ideas they have not mastered. New items are added after students have mastered previous ones. Through use of the writing checklist, students can become independent diagnosticians of their own work.

The diagnostic grid sheet is a similar record maintained by a teacher as a way of following the needs and progress of individual students. The grid sheet can cover all categories of skills to be dealt with in the curriculum. A sample diagnostic grid sheet given in the curriculum guide covers the broad categories of vocabulary development, grammatical usage, sentence structure, organization of writing, and punctuation.[23]

These grid sheet skills are tied to whole sets of suggested activities, which are sequentially organized within linguistically meaningful categories. It is not possible to do justice to this material in any brief form. The interested reader should review the Weehawken

COMMUNICATION SPIRAL

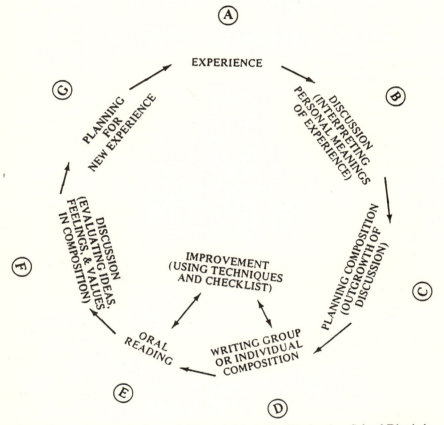

Figure 10-1. Communication activities spiral from the Weehawken School District's language arts curriculum in New Jersey. From E. Ezor, *Individual Language Arts*, 1974. Courtesy of Weehawken School District, Weehawken, New Jersey.

curriculum manual. However, brief examples will follow to convey the flavor of some types of activities.   .

In the area of vocabulary development, one of the goals is to have students use "new vocabulary words elicited in oral or writing activities, or taught in spelling, dictionary, thesaurus, or reading activities."[24] One activity in this area simply involves having students create sentences from specific vocabulary. Initially, students could be given a number of words from their sight vocabulary or oral vocabulary and be asked to make up as many sentences as they can using these sets of words. At a more advanced level, a larger number of words are given and students are asked to use the words in creating a story, letter, or poem.

In the area of grammar, one of the goals of any writing program must be to have children achieve a sense of appropriate word order at the same time as they are building more interesting and complex sentences. An activity called *slotting* is useful. In the case of noun phrases, slotting begins with a simple noun phrase drawn from the student's own interests, such as *the clown*. Then a slot is opened between the article and the noun. Children are asked to fill in the slot with any interesting word that fits.

> The_____clown
> smiling
> tall
> silly
> circus

Then a new slot can be added in front of, or in back of, the added modifer, and a second set of modifers can be created.

> The_____silly clown
> completely
> big
> tumbling
> flying

Then the order can be reversed so that a child can experiment with the order.

> The silly_____clown
> completely
> big
> tumbling
> flying

All of the variations in order should be read aloud so that a child can begin to achieve a sense of which order sounds better.

The completely silly clown

The silly completely clown

The flying silly clown
The silly flying clown

Through a series of these activities, it can be taught that noun phrases consist of elements including nouns (astronaut, ballerina), adjectives (brave, anxious), intensifiers (very, rather), qualifiers (three, many), possessives (our, her), demonstratives (this, those), and articles (an, the). Experimenting at putting together these common components of noun phrases, reading them aloud, and seeing how they sound can lead children to a richer understanding of language.

These few example exercises hardly touch the surface of the Weehawhen curriculum. The guide can be reviewed for further detail. The curriculum is compatible with the style of the spatial child, i.e. their need to be motivated by the functional and expressive value of language rather than by language for its own sake and their need to have sensitivity to language structure reinforced rather than assumed. The curriculum gives continual opportunities for real communication with others. It moves gradually from a simple, nonthreatening level to a more complex, creative level. It provides continual practice for the child rather than stressing the memorization of abstract formulations. It stresses creative production rather than rigid, boring workbook activities.

REFERENCES

1. Fadely, J.L., and Hosler, V.N. *Understanding the Alpha Child at Home and School.* Springfield, Ill.: Charles C Thomas, Publisher, 1979, p. 158.
2. *Ibid.,* pp. 157-158.
3. Bannatyne, A. *Language, Reading and Learning Disabilities.* Springfield, Ill.: Charles C Thomas, Publisher, 1971, p. 633.
4. Fadely and Hosler, *op. cit.,* p. 174.
5. Fadely and Hosler, *op. cit.,* pp. 170-171.
6. Dolch, E.W. *The Basic Sight Word List.* Champaign, Ill.: Garrard, 1972.
7. Bannatyne, *op. cit.,* p. 646.
8. Bannatyne, A. *Psycholinguistic Color System: A Reading, Writing, Spelling and Language Program.* Urbana, Ill.: Learning Systems Press, 1968.
9. Downing, J.A. *The Initial Teaching Alphabet Reading Experiment.* Chicago, Ill.: Scott, Foresman, 1964.
10. Georgiades, N.J. *Report on the Use of I.T.A. in Remedial Reading Classes.* London: Reading Research Unit, 1964.

11. Gattegno, C. *What We Owe Children: The Subordination of Teaching to Learning.* New York: Avon Books, 1971, pp. 37-42.
12. Gattegno, C. *Teaching Reading with Words-In-Color.* New York: Xerox Corporation, 1968.
13. Bannatyne, 1971, *op. cit.,* p. 667.
14. Bannatyne, 1971, *op. cit.,* p. 668.
15. Bannatyne, 1971, *op. cit.,* p. 669.
16. Fadely and Hosler, *op. cit.,* p. 177.
17. Bannatyne, 1971, *op. cit.,* p. 670.
18. Singer, J.L. *The Inner World of Daydreaming.* New York: Harper and Row, 1975.
19. Fadely and Hosler, *op. cit.,* pp. 178-179.
20. Ezor, E. *Individual Language Arts.* Weehawken, New Jersey: Weehawken School District, 1974.
21. *Ibid.,* p. 1.
22. *Ibid.,* p. 8.
23. *Ibid.,* p. 22.
24. *Ibid.,* p. 28.

Chapter 11

MEMORY

I T is well established that children who have difficulties with reading also tend to have general difficulties with memory tasks.[1] It is
also well known that people who are characteristically introverted
rather than extroverted in personality tend to have memory problems, especially in short-term memory of detailed information acquired under pressured conditions.[2] Eysenck's review of research on
this topic tends to indicate that when introverted people acquire information under less hurried, less pressured conditions, the difference tends to disappear. This might support Smith's contention that
introverted people often have a preferred information processing
mode in which they attempt to integrate new information into complex systems of previously acquired knowledge.[3] This complex integration process would debilitate the person when under pressure to
process many details quickly.

Whatever the basis for the memory problems, to the extent that
spatial children are disabled in dealing with formal language, and to
the extent that they are introverted in personality, they can also be
expected to have difficulty with remembering details. Both Alexander Bannatyne in his work with "genetic dyslexic" children and
Fadely and Hosler in their work with "alpha" children concur in this
expectation.[4]

It is part of all of our experience that making the effort to learn
something is not necessarily sufficient to assure that it will be retained in memory and be available for recall at a later time. We
learn some things that quickly fade from memory and other things
once learned seem to be available for long periods of time. There is
considerable evidence that the way we learn things in the first place
has a lot to do with how well we are able to retain them for later
recall.

One of the more conclusive findings of memory research is that
bits and pieces of limited information are more easily retained when
they are integrated into meaningful patterns of broader scopes of information.[5] In one experiment, Howe showed children pictures of

animals, explaining to them how the birth of each animal occurred.[6] At a later time, the children were asked to recall the names of the animals. Examination of the order in which the animals were recalled indicated a tendency for the animals to be grouped according to the method of birth, even though the animals had not been presented in that order. In addition, a control group of children who had not learned about the methods of birth were found to be much less effective in recalling the names of animals. Apparently, our minds spontaneously organize and interconnect information, and this is an important part of the way we are able to retain information.

Finding methods of presenting information in meaningful, connected ways is important for all children, but it is most important for spatial children. There are two techniques that can be used in this effort. One technique could be called graphics and the other imagery. There is evidence that children who are disproportionately strong in spatial ability are especially helped when information can be presented in some type of graphic representational form.[7] Kuhlman found that children who achieved higher scores on spatial testing than verbal testing are more accurate at reproducing geometric forms from memory than children having the opposite test pattern.[8] Beckman found that children who achieve higher scores on a spatial ability test benefit more than other children from learning mathematics concepts through graphic representational materials.[9] There is also evidence that children who have difficulty with formal language learning tend to be especially helped by memory techniques involving imagery.[10]

GRAPHICS

There is no set collection of methods by which any and all subject matter can be approached through graphic representation. Some areas of study are more amenable to graphics than others. Mathematics and the physical sciences are full of graphic ways of representing concepts and relationships. In elementary mathematics, manipulative materials are common. Mary Laycock and Gene Watson have provided a wide variety of ideas in their book, *The Fabric of Mathematics*.[11] In more advanced mathematics, graphic representation is sometimes essential to understanding. One could hardly approach a subject like calculus without graphic representation. It is perhaps fitting that Sir Isaac Newton, a prime example of a spatial child, was the developer of calculus. Chemists have their graphic representations for atoms, and they have structural components that can be assembled to make models of molecules.

In seeking materials for representing structure and relationships, one is not simply looking for a picture. Pictures can facilitate understanding. More valuable, however, are symbolic structural components that can be manipulated by students as a way of solidifying their understanding of the way systems of knowledge hang together. For example a bar graph of the relationship between the sizes of cities and the average number of arrests for murder per 1,000 is also a standard learnable means for representing relationships. It can be used in all sorts of situations. Thus, it is more than just a picture. It can become a method that students learn to use for increasing understanding as well as assisting in the retention of information.

Useful graphics requires some degree of flexible isomorphism. In other words, one or more characteristics of a subject matter must be symbolically represented in a manipulatable way. A bar graph provides a very simple one characteristic isomorphism: that of size or number. The size of the city can be large or small, and the number of murders can be many or few. Isomorphic models become more and more complex as they come to represent more of the characteristics of a subject area. In chemistry, a structural model of a molecule represents many characteristics all at the same time. It is a more complete representation of all parts and interactive relationships. It is, therefore, much more complex.

Whenever possible, teachers should use available methods of graphing and modeling to explain concepts to spatial children. When there is no existing method for representational graphics in a given subject area, a teacher faces a special challenge. Creative isomorphics is one method that has allowed some of the creative geniuses of history to derive their special insights. Producing new isomorphics is at the heart of unique creativity—the primary challenge of intellectual work. We cannot expect to be immediately perfected in our attempts because that is not the nature of creativity.

Nevertheless, if a teacher wishes to venture into creative isomorphic representation, three simple steps can be suggested. First, determine some of the most general characteristics and relationships in the area of study; general in the sense that these attributes could be involved in a variety of situations. By focusing on generalizable attributes, any isomorphism derived can be applied to understanding the commonalities and differences in these situations. Second, create some graphic or structural components to represent each general attribute. For each component, try to think of some structure or symbolism that seems appropriate to the attribute. Finally, encourage children to play with these components to represent various situations under study.

Let me give an example. Suppose that in a social studies class there is a unit on the European explorers (Marco Polo, Columbus, etc.). I pick social studies because graphic means for representing relationships and systems in social studies are not so common or easy to derive. Suppose further that the study begins with Marco Polo. Some of the more generalizable attributes that need to be represented in the Marco Polo story might be as follows:

1. The fact that Marco Polo's home was in one place, the countries he traveled to were in other locations, and they were considerable distances from each other.
2. The fact that the way of life of his home country was quite different from the way of life in the countries he traveled to and that this may have caused a sense of strangeness and insecurity.
3. The fact that Marco Polo had some knowledge and perspectives that may have been curiously interesting to people he met in his travels and possibly of some exchange value. The similar fact that the people he visited also had knowledge and understandings that were of interest and exchange value.
4. The fact that some of the differences between them may have been threatening to each other (religious differences, for example).

These are only four of the attributes one might focus on in the Marco Polo story. The important thing about these attributes is that they could apply to a wide variety of situations; they are generalizable. For example, they might be characteristic of a school child meeting new people in another city. The value of focusing on generalizable attributes is that once a system has been created, it can be applied to a wide variety of situations to stimulate thought about comparisons and analogies.

After the attributes have been determined, symbolisms can be created to represent each attribute. It helps to think of symbolisms that seem appropriate in some way to the thing being represented. A symbol system that could be used with the Marco Polo story is given in Figure 11-1. Whenever this kind of system is created, children should be encouraged to think of the system as something that can be manipulated and changed to make it become increasingly more appropriate to the material under study.

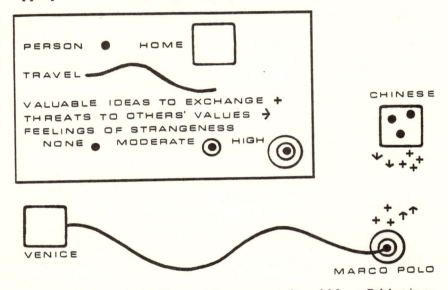

Figure 11-1. A manipulatable, symbolic representation of Marco Polo's trip to China. A generalizable system like this can be used to represent a variety of situations, such as a child visiting in a new city.

Once established, a symbol system can lead to many questions and investigations. What was the way of life in Marco Polo's home country, and what was it like in China? How different were these ways of life? Did Marco Polo feel very much out of place in China? If not, might it be more appropriate to diagram him in a different way? What were the ideas that Marco Polo exchanged with the Chinese? In what ways might the way of life of the Chinese have seemed threatening to Marco Polo and vice versa? The Chinese seemed to have been very hospitable toward Marco Polo. Might there have been circumstances under which they would have been less hospitable? Was

Marco Polo a special kind of person who could feel comfortable wherever he went? These questions might lead all the way to neuro-psychological investigations of the adrenalin fight-or-flight response to new stimuli. Might the explorers have been a special breed of people who had very low levels of sympathetic nervous system response to changes in their environment? Might children be able to find material in the biographical information on explorers that would indicate this? How could the symbol system be changed to represent physical variations of this sort?

After a group of children has explored these ideas, searched in the literature for answers to questions, and played around at adjusting the diagram according to new knowledge gained, the diagram becomes a convenient device for recalling ideas and facts from memory. If you could imagine yourself closing this book right now and writing an essay about Marco Polo in China, I think you would admit that a quick reconstruction of the diagram before you started writing would lead you to write a richer, more interesting essay. If you were a person who has difficulty retaining disconnected facts in memory, the diagram would be especially helpful to you.

Isomorphic diagrams can also encourage thinking about relationships. For example there might be some implication in the Marco Polo diagram that the further one is from home, the more one will feel out of place with cultures encountered. However, is this true? A child might realize that although Australia and Indonesia may be approximately the same distance from the United States, a child from the United States might feel somewhat more out of place in Indonesia than in Australia. Why? The answer to this question might lead to suggestions that the diagram needs to be adjusted to account for cultural similarities and differences and to account for the migration of substantial populations across long distances. A symbolism might be created that differentiates social distance from physical distance.

The further one goes in raising questions about the adequacy of the diagramming system and in making creative adjustments in it, the more a variety of ideas and facts get hung together by the diagram, and the more one is encouraged to raise more creative questions about a variety of situations and relationships. The diagram becomes both an aid to analysis and an aid to memory. Efficient memory devices involve a combination of the two intellectual processes.

I created this example because isomorphic diagramming is not common in the social sciences. I hope it demonstrates that graphic aides to memory are possible in a variety of subject areas, not just in natural science and mathematics, where there is a long tradition of graphics to rely on. It is important to use graphics as a flexible, evolving system of interacting parts, not as a rigid, pictorial given. For children to construct the graphics themselves is an important part of learning the relationships, thinking about them creatively, and holding them in memory.

IMAGERY

Mental imagery is one of the oldest and most effective means for assisting memory. Imagery techniques have been traced to the ancient Greeks who used these devices as early as the sixth century B.C. Cicero wrote of these techniques: "Persons desiring to train this faculty must select places and form mental images of the things they wish to remember and store these images in the places, so that the order of the places will preserve the order of the things and the images of the things will denote themselves."[12]

One of the most consistent findings of recent research on memory is that people are most helped by imagery that is interactive.[13] If a person were learning to associate the words *dog* and *broom* (for what weird reason I don't know), then it would be more efficient to create an image of a dog sweeping with a broom than to have images of the two separate objects. Although it is known that some people have very intense picture-like imagery of everything they have ever seen and that this gives them an extreme memory for details, static picture-like images are not helpful to more profound intellectual thought. The Russian neuropsychologist, Luria, studied the abilities of a person who possessed unusual picture-like memory and found the person to be debilitated for intellectual work. The ever-present static images made "abstract thought virtually impossible for him."[14]

A more flexible, interactive imagery is required for true intellectual work. It is known that many chess champions have phenomenal memories for play action in chess — so phenomenal that many can play blindfolded with little detriment to their ability. But their memory is not a static, picture-like memory. It is a very complex, interactive abstract imagery. Binet, in a study of chess champions, found this to be the essential difference between their imagery of chess and the imagery of less able chess players: "The experienced player leaves the concrete visual image of the chessboard to the mere amateur; to put it mildly, such a view is useless and naive. In general, the good player depends surely on abstract memory."[15] Eysenck's comment on this observation is interesting: "Obviously, the retrieval of information would be extremely difficult if storage usually consisted of highly specific, uninterpreted images. The attempted retrieval of information about one of the events of the day with such a storage system would be analogous to trying to find one specific photograph in a trunk of randomly distributed photographs."[16]

The need for an abstracted mental imagery in order to carry out higher level spatial thought processes may very well relate to Sir Francis Galton's unexpected results on the "breakfast-table" imagery study mentioned in Chapter 3. When Galton asked some of his scientifically accomplished friends to describe the vividness, the details, and the coloring in their images of their breakfast table, he found that they were rather deficient in this picture-like imagery. Higher level spatial–mechanical thought processes seem to involve abstracted, manipulative imagery similar to that described by Einstein: "Signs and more or less clear images which can be voluntarily reproduced and combined . . . to arrive finally at logically connected concepts . . . combinatory play . . . visual and some muscular type."[17]

This manipulative imagery is exactly the element most characteristic of spatial ability. Spatial manipulations are rather distinct from static pictorial imagery. This distinction is echoed by Eysenck: "Tests of spatial ability typically involve complex manipulations of imaginal processing, and this may differ from the rather simpler forms of imaginal processing."[18] Research has clearly supported the contention that picture-like imagery is not the same as the more abstract, manipulative imagery involved in spatial ability.[19]

In working with spatial children, it is especially important to take advantage of the information retrieval capacities of manipulative imagery.[20] The capacity of manipulative imagery is, perhaps, demonstrated in a research study by Morris and Stevens. They asked people to recall lists of words. In one group people were asked to link three words together into a connective image. Another group was asked to use a separate image for each word. A third group was given no special instructions on how to memorize the words. The group using linking imagery was able to recall a much larger portion of the words than the other groups.[21]

The crucial element in this linking process is to find meaningful connections between different pieces of information. If we are to take Einstein's description of his imagery as a lead, we would be working toward imagery akin to interrelated graphics described in the previous section of this chapter. We can teach children to take separate pieces of information in a topic area and to connect them into meaningful images. After this has been accomplished, the interconnectedness of the imagery causes the various parts to imply each other. The connecting conceptualizations in the imagery allow for easy reconstruction of the image in mind, and this allows for easy recall of all details.

REFERENCES

1. Berger, N.S., and Perfetti, C.A. Reading skill and memory for spoken and written discourse. *Journal of Reading Behavior, 9*:7–16, 1977; Pelham, W.E., and Ross, A.O. Selective attention in children with reading problems: a developmental study of incidental learning. *Journal of Abnormal Child Psychology, 5*: 1–8, 1977; Prawat, R.S., and Kerasotes, D. Basic memory processes in reading. *Merrill–Palmer Quarterly, 24*:181–188, 1978; Tarver, S.G., Hallahan, D.P., Kauffman, J.M., and Ball, D.W. Verbal rehearsal and selective attention in children with learning disabilities: a developmental lag. *Journal of Experimental Child Psychology, 22*:375–385, 1976; Torgesen, J.K. Memorization processes in reading-disabled children. *Journal of Educational Psychology, 69*:571–578, 1977; Wong, B., Wong, R., and Foth, D. Recall and clustering of verbal materials among normal and poor readers. *Bulletin of the Psychonomic Society, 10*:375–378, 1977.

2. Eysenck, M.W. *Human Memory: Theory, Research and Individual Differences.* Oxford: Pergamon Press, 1977, pp. 202–208.

3. Smith, I.M. *Spatial Ability: Its Educational and Social Significance.* London: University of London Press, 1964, p. 291.

4. Bannatyne, A. *Language, Reading and Learning Disabilities.* Springfield, Ill.: Charles C Thomas, Publisher, 1971, p. 690; Fadely, J.L., and Hosler, V.N. *Understanding the Alpha Child at Home and School.* Springfield, Ill.: Charles C Thomas, Publisher, 1979, pp. 180–184.

5. Bower, G.H. Imagery as a relational organizer in associative learning. *Journal of Verbal Learning and Verbal Behavior, 9*:529–533, 1970; Higbee, K.L. Recent research on visual mnemonics: historical roots and educational fruits. *Review of*

Educational Research, 49:616–617, 1979.

6. Howe, M.J.A., and Ceci, S.J. Educational implications of memory research. In Gruneberg, M.M, and Morris, P.E. *Applied Problems in Memory*. London: Academic Press, 1979, p. 74.

7. Stewart, J.C. *An Experimental Investigation of Imagery*. Unpublished Ph.D. thesis, University of Toronto, 1965.

8. Kuhlman, C.K. *Visual Imagery in Children*. Unpublished Ph.D. thesis, Radcliffe College, 1960.

9. Beckman, L. Use of the block design sub-test of the WISC as an instrument for identifying children who prefer a non-verbal (spatial) approach to learning. In Gallagher, J. *Gifted Children: Reaching Their Potential*. Jerusalem: Kollek and Son, Ltd., 1979.

10. Jorm, A.F. Effect of word imagery on reading performance as a function of reader ability. *Journal of Educational Psychology, 69*:46–54, 1977; Torgesen, *op. cit.*, pp. 571–578.

11. Laycock, M., and Watson, G. *The Fabric of Mathematics*. Hayward, Calif.: Activity Resources Company, 1975.

12. Higbee, *op. cit.*, pp. 611–629.

13. Higbee, *op. cit.*, p. 617; Eysenck, *op. cit.*, p. 44

14. Howe and Ceci, *op. cit.*, p. 67.

15. Binet, A. Mnemonic virtuosity: a study of chess players. *Genetic Psychological Monographs, 74*:127–162, 1966.

16. Eysenck, *op. cit.*, p. 52

17. Einstein, A. Letter to Jacques Hadamard. In Ghiselin, B. *The Creative Process*. New York: Mentor Books, 1952, p. 43.

18. Eysenck, *op. cit.*, p. 277

19. DiVeste, F.J., Ingersoll, G., and Sunshine, P. A factor analysis of imagery tests. *Journal of Verbal Learning and Verbal Behavior, 10*:471–479, 1971.

20. Hollenberg, C.K. Functions of visual imagery in the learning and concept formation of children. *Child Development, 41*:1003–1015, 1970; Klee, H., and Eysenck, M.W. Comprehension of abstract and concrete sentences. *Journal of Verbal Learning and Verbal Behavior, 12*:522–529, 1972.

21. Morris, P.E., and Stevens, R. Linking images and free recall. *Journal of Verbal Learning and Verbal Behavior, 13*:310–315, 1974.

INDEX